Nutrition and Cancer

CURRENT CONCEPTS IN NUTRITION

Myron Winick, Editor

Institute of Human Nutrition
Columbia University College of Physicians and Surgeons

Volume 1: Nutrition and Development
Volume 2: Nutrition and Fetal Development
Volume 3: Childhood Obesity
Volume 4: Nutrition and Aging
Volume 5: Nutritional Disorders of American Women
Volume 6: Nutrition and Cancer

NUTRITION AND CANCER

Edited by

MYRON WINICK

Institute of Human Nutrition
Columbia University College of Physicians and Surgeons

A WILEY-INTERSCIENCE PUBLICATION

JOHN WILEY & SONS
New York • **Chichester** • **Brisbane** • **Toronto**

Library of Congress Cataloging in Publication Data:

Nutrition and cancer.

  (Current concepts in nutrition; v. 6)
  "A Wiley-Interscience publication."
    1. Cancer—Nutritional aspects.   I. Winick, Myron.
II. Series. [DNLM: 1. Diet—Adverse effects.
2. Neoplasms—Etiology. 3. Neoplasms—Prevention and
control.   W1 CU788AS v. 6 / QZ202 N976]
RC262.N87   616.9′94   77-22650

ISBN 0-471-03394-4

Printed in the United States of America

10 9 8 7 6 5 4 3 2 1

Contents

PART 3   PREVENTION AND THERAPY

Nutrition and Cancer

Introduction

MYRON WINICK, M.D.

Institute of Human Nutrition, College of Physicians and Surgeons,
Columbia University, New York, New York

Nutrition is involved in at least three aspects of the cancer problem. As Dr. Paul Marks, Director of Columbia Medical School's Cancer Research Center, points out in his introductory chapter nutrition is important in the etiology of cancer. Cancer itself and certain forms of cancer therapy may profoundly affect the nutritional status of a patient and research is beginning to suggest that certain kinds of nutritional manipulations may play an important part in the treatment of certain types of cancer.

This volume is an attempt to organize our knowledge in these three areas and to examine critically what is known, what remains to be learned, and what are the most promising directions for future research. In addition, wherever feasible, practical recommendations for patient management are made.

The book is divided into three parts: Nutrition and the Cause of Cancer; Nutrient Deficiencies; Prevention and Therapy. After the overview by Dr. Marks, the first part continues with a discussion of nutrition and experimental carcinogenesis by David B. Clayson. Total dietary restriction or specifically limiting carbohydrate intake has been shown to reduce the incidence of certain tumors in mice and rats. By contrast, limiting the protein content of the diet generally had very little effect on overall incidence of most tumors. Both the quantity and the quality of dietary fat can influence tumor incidence. Deficiency in lipotropes results in an increased incidence of both spontaneous and induced liver tumors in rats and chickens. Although results are not conclusive it has been suggested that vitamin A and vitamin C may protect against certain types of tumors. Finally, the timing of a dietary stress has been shown to be extremely important. An increasing body of evidence suggests that nutritional manipulations early in life—even in the preweaning period—may alter the incidence of spontaneously occurring tumors and affect ultimate longevity in rats.

1

Dr. K. K. Carroll discusses the induction of mammary tumors in animals by fat in the diet. He points out that unsaturated fat is a more potent stimulus to tumor genesis than saturated fat. In addition, he postulates that fat acts as a promoting agent, enhancing the potency of certain carcinogens, rather than as a carcinogen itself. These data in rats are reinforced by studies in humans, which demonstrate a strong positive correlation between dietary fat intake and age-adjusted mortality from breast cancer in different countries of the world. Similar but somewhat weaker correlations have been observed between fat intake and certain other types of cancer, including prostatic cancer and ovarian cancer.

The association of high dietary fat and low fiber intake with carcinoma of the colon is discussed in the chapters by Drs. Wynder and Kritchevsky. They discuss the fact that tumors of the large bowel can be related to several dietary components. Thus, there is a positive correlation between bowel cancer mortality and dietary fat consumption. It has also been stated that there is an inverse correlation between incidence of bowel cancer and dietary fiber. Populations ingesting a Western-style high fat diet ingest little fiber and the question of which component is truly responsible for the observed correlations has not been answered.

Proponents of the high fiber hypothesis suggest that the more rapid transit time which results from such diets reduces the duration of contact between exogenous carginogens and the tissue. Support has been lent to the high fat hypothesis by findings of differences in the spectra of neutral and acidic fecal steroids between animals with induced colon cancer and controls. The transformations in fecal steroids are, in large part, a product of the action of intestinal microorganisms. The question then becomes, which influences the spectrum of intestinal flora, fat or fiber? This critical point is far from resolution and data that tend to support both arguments are presented.

Part 2 is concerned with nutrient deficiencies caused by various types of cancer. The problem of cancer cachexia is discussed by Athanasios Theologides. He points out that cachexia occurs in one-third to two-thirds of cancer patients. It is characterized by anorexia, increased basal metabolic rate and energy expenditure despite the reduced caloric intake, marked asthenia, loss of body fat, protein, and other components, anemia, and water and electrolyte disturbances. Although the anorexia leads to reduced food intake, the weight loss can be stopped only temporarily by increasing that intake even with measures such as hyperalimentation. Thus it is the cancer growth itself that contributes to the cachectic syndrome, either by successfully competing for available nutrients or by deranging the host metabolism in some way.

A common finding in patients with cancer bis hypoalbuminemia. Dr. Thomas Waldman has demonstrated that this condition is often caused by a decrease in the synthesis of albumin. In addition, however, certain types of cancer result in an excessive loss of proteins into the gastrointestinal tract. This loss may occur in patients with carcinoma of the stomach or with carinoid tumors of the gastrointestinal tract. Finally, patients with lymphosarcoma or Hodgkin's disease may lose lymphocyte-rich lymph into the gut.

Another recent observation is that patients with various types of cancer may exhibit a variety of vitamin deficiencies. Dr. John Dickerson has observed low plasma levels of vitamin A in patients with advanced disease of the alimentary tract and with squamous and oat cell carcinoma of the lung. Certain patients with lung and breast cancer, especially those being treated with 5-fluorouracil, showed a low thiamin status and high values of thiamin pyrophosphate (TPP). The data suggest an abnormality in thiamin metabolism rather than a dietary deficiency.

In patients with breast cancer and skeletal metastasis low levels of leukocyte ascorbic acid and high levels of urinary hydroxyproline (OHP) were observed. Supplementation with ascorbic acid reduced the OHP excretion within four hours.

These data suggest that in patients with cancer at certain sites the requirements for specific vitamins may be changed and therefore that attention to these changed requirements might be useful in the management of the patient.

Part 3 deals with prevention and therapy of cancer using nutritional means. One of the newest and potentially most exciting approaches to cancer prevention has been the use of vitamin A analogs in experimental animals to prevent the induction of epithelial tumors of the bronchi, trachea, stomach, uterus, and skin. Dr. Michael Sporn points out that these studies, while currently in the experimental stage, are potentially important in a variety of human populations—most notably where precancerous lesions can be identified and where a high risk for cancer is present.

Dr. William DeWys discusses the problem of anorexia and more specifically abnormalities of taste in the cancer patient. In a series of studies, he has demonstrated that patients with limited disease generally had normal taste sensation. By contrast, patients with widespread disease generally showed marked abnormalities in taste. In addition, when treatment has been successful in reducing the size of the tumor, taste perception has returned to normal. These observations may be of value in the management of anorectic cancer patients. Patients with an elevated threshold for sweet taste may be able to increase their food intake if they increase the seasoning on their food. In patients with a low bitter threshold, there often is a range of preference related to protein source, with beef and pork being less desirable, poultry and fish intermediate, and cheese and eggs often remaining pleasurable.

Dr. Sarah Donaldson describes the consequences of radiation therapy and the use of certain cytotoxic drugs that lead to anorexia, weight loss, and malnutrition. This malnutrition is not only damaging to the patient but may prevent an aggressive therapeutic approach to the patient's primary condition. Dr. Maurice Shils describes the use of special diets for supporting patients, for rehabilitating patients who have been treated successfully, and for preparing patients for various forms of therapy. One method that is being used more frequently is total parenteral nutrition (TPN) using a central venous catheter.

Dr. Shils also discusses how TPN therapy is administered, which patients can most benefit from the use of TPN, and some of the specific indications and contraindications for this form of treatment.

The area of nutrition and cancer is just beginning to receive the attention it should. I would expect much to be learned in the near future. This volume has very few definitive answers. That is not its purpose. Instead, it summarizes what little is known and charts some new directions for the future.

PART 1

Nutrition and the Cause of Cancer

1

Nutrition and the Cancer Problem

PAUL A. MARKS

Cancer Research Center, Columbia University, New York City

The role of diet is gaining prominence in the investigation of why some people get cancer and others do not. For many years evidence has accumulated that a number of diseases in addition to cancer, such as heart disease, diabetes, arthritis, and dental caries, are related to diet (1). Although there are many clues that associate these diseases with dietary excesses or deficiencies, there is no definitive scientific evidence that any of these chronic diseases is caused by dietary factors alone. Recently an increasing number of studies have related dietary and nutrient excesses, deficiencies, or imbalances to the development of cancers in the esophagus, stomach, colon, pancreas, liver, and breast (2).

Diet and nutrition are of interest not only as determinants of carcinogenesis, that is, of susceptibility or resistance to cancer development. Investigation is also needed to define more precisely the role of diet and nutrition as an adjunct to other therapeutic modalities, such as surgery, radiotherapy, chemotherapy, and immunotherapy, and to discover the role of specific nutritional manipulation in the prevention and therapy of certain cancers.

NUTRITION AND THE CAUSATION OF CANCERS

The suspicion that nutrition may be involved in the cause of cancer has derived primarily from epidemiological studies and a number of animal laboratory studies. It is estimated that over one-half of all female cancer deaths and 30% of all male cancer deaths may be related to nutritional factors (3). This estimate does not include accidental or intentional food

7

additives that may be carcinogenic. This accumulating evidence suggests that many of the common types of cancer may be caused in part by nutritional factors. Because we can act to alter nutrition, these cancers are potentially avoidable.

The group most conspicuously at risk for cancer is, of course, the elderly. Various models have been proposed to account for clustering of cancer in old age. One reasonable theory of carcinogenesis states that in each cell there are several genes that function independently to prevent cancerous transformation, and that cancer will not occur until each of these genes has been inactivated by mutation. Since a mutation can be introduced in the genome at any time during the life of a cell or of its ancestors, the chances of inactivating all the cancer-preventing genes increase directly with age. This theory predicts that the log of cancer

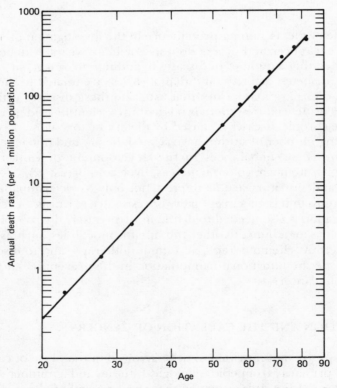

Figure 1. Relationship between age (years) and mortality from all forms of cancer (annual death rate expressed per 1 million population). Reprinted from Carins (4) with permission.

incidence should be linearly related to the log of our age. In fact this relation of incidence to age is observed for a number of cancers (4) (Fig. 1).

This relationship between age and incidence of cancer has several important implications for our consideration of nutrition as a causal factor in cancer. First, it suggests that a given cancer may have several factors contributing to its cause. Second, a cancer may be the end result of several events occurring over a period of a person's life; in other words, we may have to look to the nutritional environment of the early life of an individual to understand the role of dietary factors in the causation of cancer. Various studies of migrant populations suggest that the incidence of certain common cancers may be partly determined by our nutritional habits in youth. Third, the other side of the argument is that potentially it could take many years before an increased incidence of a particular cancer calls attention to the danger of dietary factors.

Many population studies now provide rather convincing evidence that environment, and possibly nutrition, play decisive roles in the causation of cancer. For example, cancer of the stomach is much more common in Japan than in the United States, but cancer of the large intestine, breast, and prostate are much less common (5). Further, there is a change in incidence of various cancers with migration from Japan to the United States (5–7) (Fig. 2). This suggests that cancers are caused by environmental factors that differ in the two countries. The death rates among Japanese immigrants and immigrants' sons tend consistently toward California norms, but the change requires more than one generation. Therefore some of the causative agents must be factors such as diet, which tend to persist as part of a cultural heritage, rather than factors such as air pollution, which tend to be the same for everyone in a given area.

Similar observations have been made among Jewish populations who migrated to Israel from Europe or the United States (8). The immigrants from Europe or the United States have an incidence of cancer that is typical of their country of origin, but their children, born in Israel, have a much lower incidence of almost all kinds of cancers. In this respect they become more like the indigenous Israeli population and like Jewish immigrants from Asia and Africa.

The incidence of cancer of the large intestine among women in 23 countries is closely related to per capita meat consumption in these countries (9–11) (Fig. 3). An alternative nutritional explanation of these data, put forth by various investigators, is that in areas of high incidence of colon cancers, the diet consumed tends to be high in refined foods and low in unabsorbed cellulose or fiber. Differences in bacterial flora as-

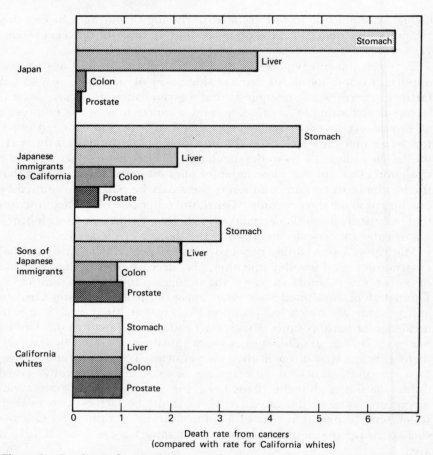

Figure 2. Death rate from various types of cancers among Japanese and Japanese immigrants to California, compared with California whites. Reprinted from Cairns (4) with permission.

sociated with the two types of diet have been documented. There are other studies in progress employing in vitro assays for mutagenesis, attempting to identify specific substances in feces and in urine which are mutagenic and possibly carcinogenic.

In this book several investigators in this field will discuss in detail other studies which persuade us that there is a relationship between neoplasia and dietary practices.

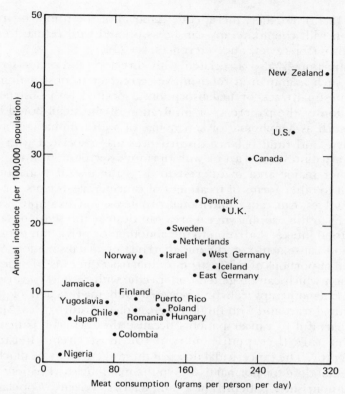

Figure 3. Relationship between incidence of cancer of the large intestine among women in 23 countries and meat consumption expressed as grams per person per day. Reprinted from Cairns (4) with permission.

NUTRITIONAL STATUS AND TREATMENT OF THE PATIENT WITH CANCER

The effects of cancer on the nutritional status of the patient are another important subject to be discussed. The striking and still poorly understood effect of cancer is the marked anorexia associated with a number of neoplasms. Several studies document effects on nitrogen balance, carbohydrate tolerance, and insulin sensitivity which indicate that in patients with cancer there may be abnormalities in metabolism which cannot be explained on the basis of the tumor mass or of the dietary intake (12,13). Further, therapeutic removal of the tumor or inducing remission with chemotherapy can be associated with return to normal metabolism (for review and references, see (14).

Malnutrition is also associated with direct or indirect effects of a cancer, such as impaired food intake secondary to obstruction of the gastrointestinal tract, or malabsorption associated with obstruction or destruction of the pancreas, or infiltration of the small bowel by neoplasms such as lymphomas or carcinoma, or with lymphatic obstruction. Electrolyte and fluid balance disturbances are associated with tumors in the gastrointestinal tract or with hormone-secreting tumors.

Another major area of interest to us is the use of nutrition as an adjuvant to other forms of treatment of cancer. Treatments for cancer, in themselves, can cause nutritional problems. For example, radiation treatment to the oropharyngeal area can destroy the sense of taste and impair food intake. Radiation to the abdomen or pelvis can damage the bowel and cause acute or chronic diarrhea or malabsorption. Surgical resection of portions of the gastrointestinal tract can cause deficiencies in absorption which can be general or specific with respect to various nutrients. Chemotherapy can be associated with malfunction of the gastrointestinal tract and with fluid and electrolyte disturbances. Malnutrition is harmful to cancer patients because the cachectic patient has a narrower safe therapeutic margin for most chemotherapy and radiotherapy. The cancericidal doses of these agents may be much closer to the lethal dose for normal tissues in the malnourished patient than in the well-nourished patient. For example, Drs. Edward Copeland and Stanley J. Dudrick (15) and others have provided evidence that the application of intravenous hyperalimentation to the treatment of cancer patients is safe, tumor growth is not stimulated, and chemotherapy and radiotherapy are better tolerated. This is an area where more detailed evaluation of the nutritional values and protocols for nutrient administration should be of great benefit in therapy and rehabilitation of cancer patients.

NUTRITIONAL MANIPULATION AS THERAPY FOR CANCER

An exciting area of investigation has been opened with the observation that nutritional manipulation per se may be an approach to treatment of certain cancers. For example, an approach to chemoprevention of forms of epithelial cancer during the period of preneoplasia has been reported with the finding that vitamin A and its synthetic analogs, the retinoids, are potent agents for control of cell differentiation in several epithelial tissues (16). In experimental animals, deficiency of dietary retinoids enhances susceptibility to chemical carcinogenesis. Synthetic retinoids have been made which are active in moderating the effects of polycyclic hydrocarbons as inducers of epithelial cancers in animals.

Evidence that nutrition plays a role in cancer causation is strongly supported by epidemiological studies and by certain studies on animals. There is clearly a need for major research emphasis to further define the role of dietary components as determinants of carcinogenesis in man. In the area of therapy, we sorely need to increase our understanding of the role of diet as an adjuvant to existing therapy and of methods to deal with the altered nutrient metabolism associated with neoplasia. Last, but far from least, investigations of the role of nutritional manipulation may provide important new approaches to the prevention and therapy of cancer.

REFERENCES

1. R. S. Goodhart and M. E. Shils, *Modern Nutrition in Health and Disease*, 5th Ed., Lea and Febiger, Philadelphia (1973) p. 1153.

2. Symposium on Nutrition in the Causation of Cancer, *Cancer Res.*, **35** (Part 2), 3231–3550 (1975).

3. G. B. Gori and E. Wynder, Contribution of the environment ot cancer incidence: Epidemiologic exercise. *J. Natl Cancer Insti.*, in press.

4. J. Carins, *Sci. Amer.*, **233**, 64 (1975).

5. J. E. Dunn, *Cancer Res.*, **35**, 3240 (1975).

6. W. Haenszel and M. Kurihara, *J. Natl. Cancer Inst.*, **40**, 43 (1968).

7. P. Buell and J. E. Dunn, *Cancer*, **18**, 656 (1965).

8. R. Doll, C. Muir and J. Waterhouse, Eds., *Cancer Incidence in Five Continents*, Vol. 2, International Union Against Cancer, Springer-Verlag, New York (1970).

9. B. Armstrong and R. Doll, *Intl. J. Cancer*, **15**, 617 (1975).

10. M. J. Hill, *Cancer Res.*, **35**, 3398 (1975).

11. E. L. Wynder, *Cancer Res.*, **35**, 3388 (1975).

12. P. A. Marks and J. S. Bishop, *J. Clin. Invest.*, **36,** 254 (1957).

13. J. S. Bishop and P. A. Marks, *J. Clin. Invest.*, **38**, 668 (1959).

14. M. E. Shils, "Nutrition and Neoplasia," *in* R. S. Goodhart and M. E. Shils, Eds., *Modern Nutrition in Health and Disease*, 5th Ed., Lea and Febiger, Philadelphia (1973), p. 981.

15. E. M. Copeland and S. J. Dudrick, *Current Problems in Cancer*, **1**, 1 (1976).

16. M. D. Sporn, N. M. Dunlop, D. L. Newton and J. M. Smith, *Fed. Proc.*, **35**, 1332 (1976).

2

Nutrition and Experimental Carcinogenesis

DAVID B. CLAYSON

Eppley Institute for Research in Cancer, University of Nebraska Medical Center, Omaha, Nebraska

Experimental studies of nutritional variables and their effect on cancer induction in laboratory animals will be discussed in this chapter. The effect of changes in calorie intake, of the level and type of fat consumed, and similar alterations will be considered. The equally fascinating and important topic of the possible action of man-made food additives or natural food contaminants is largely outside our present discussion.

Epidemiological and experimental studies represent the two major bases for our present attitudes toward environmental carcinogenesis. The two areas are complementary, and to establish firm conclusions, both are necessary. Epidemiological studies in man deal with highly heterogenous populations and rely heavily on statistical methods to draw conclusions from a mass of often uncontrolled and uncontrollable variables. Animal studies, on the other hand, concern relatively strictly controlled populations with the minimum attainable number of variables, but, unfortunately, present considerable difficulties when extrapolation is made across species to man.

ANIMAL EXPERIMENTATION

The major restriction on animal experiments in nutrition and carcinogenesis studies is cost. In animals, tumors take a considerable portion of the lifespan to develop, which means that even with shorter-lived

Supported by Public Health Service Contract NO1 CP33278 from the Division of Cancer Cause and Prevention, the National Cancer Institute, National Institutes of Health.

animals, such as rats, mice, and hamsters, the experimental period may last from 1 to 3 years. Costs are therefore high, if an adequate number of animals is to be attained to permit proper statistical evaluation of the results. Supervision of the animals' diet, using such methods as "pair-feeding" to ensure that experimental and control groups are truly equivalent, considerably increases the labor required to conduct experiments and thereby inflates the cost. As it is now realized that dietary modification has the potential to alter the site, as well as the number, of tumors, all experiments directed toward elucidation of effects of nutrition and cancer require a full autopsy. The autopsy should be conducted by technicians familiar with the appearance of gross pathological changes, which may result from dietary modification. Also, professionals should prepare and examine histological slides to clearly establish the nature of any changes.

Nutritional variations may affect the developmental stage of the tumor, or in the case of chemical carcinogens, the conversion of a relatively stable precarcinogen to its highly reactive (electrophilic) form (1). It is especially desirable to determine which stage of tumorigenesis is being affected because conversion to an active form is now known to differ between species, whereas developmental phenomena, such as cell proliferation, immunocompetence, and hormone levels, may show greater trans-species similarities. For this reason, it is important, where possible, to give a chemical carcinogen once, or for a limited time, and then to await tumor development. The effects of nutritional variations on both phases may then be elucidated independently.

EXPERIMENTAL RESULTS OF NUTRITIONAL MODIFICATION

Calorie Restriction

Tannenbaum (2) consulted actuarial records from insurance companies and concluded that the overweight or obese were somewhat more at risk from cancer than normal or underweight people. This led to a series of nutritional experiments, mainly in mice, which, although the work is 20 to 30 years old, still represent the best available data in this area. Dietary restriction reduced the incidence of mammary tumor, virus-induced breast tumors in DBA and C_3H mice, spontaneous lung tumors in Swiss and ABC mice benzo(a)pyrene (B(a)P)-induced skin tumors, and, to a lesser extent, subcutaneous sarcomas induced by B(a)P (3, 4). Similar effects have been observed in rats. As in mice, underfeeding greatly increased the lifespan and led to a lower tumor incidence than that in animals receiving *ad libitum* food (5 - 7). In these underfeeding studies, the amounts of the various dietary components were reduced proportionately to each other.

An alternative to underfeeding is calorie restriction, in which the amount of carbohydrate (i.e., starches and sugars) is reduced, while other components are maintained at a constant level. Calorie-restricted diets again lessen the incidence or delay the appearance of certain neoplasms, such as mammary tumors in DBA mice (4). The inhibition was apparent, even if the restricted diet was instituted when the mice were nine months old, that is to say, some three to six months before tumors began to appear in those fed *ad libitum*.

The mechanism by which dietary restriction inhibits tumorigenesis is unknown. Initiation-promotion studies in skin carcinogenesis showed that restriction was effective in the promotion or developmental stage of tumor formation, but some influence on the initiation stage could not be excluded by the data presented (8).

The body weight or some reflection of it, rather than the number of calories consumed, seems to be the key factor, since mice fed a thyroid supplement consumed a considerable excess of calories, but did not gain in body weight or alter their tumor incidence (9). These classic experiments and others of a similar nature clearly demonstrate the importance of calorie intake and body weight on the level of both naturally occurring and induced tumors. Nutritional experiments are valueless when they ignore the necessity of balancing the body weight of each experimental group of test animals.

Protein

The feeding of isocaloric diets containing protein levels ranging from 9 to 45% influenced neither the incidence of mammary tumors in DBA and C_3H mice, nor the incidence of hydrocarbon-induced skin tumors and subcutaneous sarcomas (10). Spontaneous hepatomas in C_3H mice occurred less frequently when the 9% protein diet was fed. This was due to a diminution in the concentration of the essential sulfur-containing amino acids, cysteine and methionine (c.f., "lipotrope deficiency"). The addition of sufficient protein free of these amino acids to raise the protein level from 9% to 18%, failed to affect the incidence of spontaneous hepatomas, whereas addition of the calculated amounts of these amino acids did so (11).

High protein levels protect the rat liver against carcinogenesis by the azo dye 4-dimethylaminoazobenzene. Adequate dietary casein, even with low levels of riboflavin, also protects the rat liver against this chemical (12). The reason for this phenomenon is not known. Tannenbaum and Silverstone suggested that the high protein diet might be protective because it enabled the liver to store and utilize riboflavin more efficiently.

Ross and Bras (13) more recently reported on feeding diets containing 10, 22, or 51% casein on either a restricted (equicaloric) or an *ad libitum* regimen to rats. Longevity increased from the group of rats fed 10% casein *ad libitum* to that fed 51% casein restricted, and tended to increase with the amount of protein in the diet in the *ad libitum* groups. The most common tumor in the high protein groups was papilloma of the urinary bladder. Urinary stone formation was not described (14). Possibly, this is an effect of an increased amount of the essential amino acid tryptophan administered in the high protein diet. It has been suggested that the urinary output of those tryptophan metabolites on the niacin pathway is higher in some patients with nonoccupational bladder cancer than in normal subjects (15). Furthermore, feeding a sevenfold excess of DL-tryptophan to dogs led to hyperplasia of the urinary bladder (16). An increase in the proliferation of the rat bladder epithelium has also been reported on a similar regimen. The metabolites of tryptophan responsible for these effects have not been positively identified.

Very low levels of protein affect the way the body handles carcinogens. Thus, dimethylnitrosamine (DMN) is acutely hepatotoxic to rats maintained on a basal diet, but less so if the rats are maintained on a special protein-free diet (17). This is of interest in experiments in which tumors are induced by a single dose of DMN. Hepatotoxicity kills rats given a single large dose of this chemical. With a protein-free diet fed for 8 to 10 days around the time a single dose of DMN is administered, followed by the basal diet for the rest of the animals' life, a greatly enhanced incidence of kidney tumors is obtained, because the low protein diet protects the liver, enabling a greater dose of chemical to be given, and thus more carcinogen to reach the kidney.

Lipotrope Deficiency

Lipotropic substances are those which prevent or correct fatty liver due to choline deficiency. Lipotrope-deficient diets are low in choline and methionine. Choline-deficient diets *per se* in rats and chickens surviving beyond 78 weeks led to fatty livers and to liver tumors (18, 19). More recent confirmation of these results is lacking, and the possibility cannot be excluded that the liver tumors were a consequence of the interaction of the hepatotoxic diet and adventitious contamination with a natural carcinogen, such as aflatoxin B_1. There is evidence that lipotrope-deficient diets enhance hepatocarcinogenesis by B_1, diethylnitrosamine (DEN) and dibutylnitrosamine (20–22). Esophageal cancer induction by DEN was possibly also enhanced. Other tumors were not affected. The lipotrope-deficient diets have been demonstrated to reduce the activity of hepatic metabolizing enzymes, such as aminopyrene demethylase, p-nitroaniline demethylase, and $B(a)P$ hydroxylase and also to increase the mitotic rate in the liver (21, 22).

Lipids

Lipids are of great interest at this time as possible factors in the causation of human breast and colon cancer. It is not clear whether they act as nutritional modifiers of the carcinogenic process, perhaps in a way similar to caloric restriction, or whether they are vehicles for the transport of other carcinogens into the body. Experimental work does not give much support so far to their importance in carcinogenesis.

The high caloric value of fat makes it essential to feed equicaloric amounts of each diet. Tannenbaum (23) showed, by using equicaloric diets, that a regimen containing enhanced levels of fat increased the incidence of $B(a)P$-induced skin tumors in Swiss, C57 Black, and DBA mice, and of naturally occurring hepatomas in C_3H mice. With mammary tumors in DBA mice, either the latency was reduced or the number of tumors increased. There was no effect on subcutaneous sarcoma or lung adenoma induction. The positive affects were of a lower order than those seen with caloric restriction, which led to the suggestion that they may have been due to different "energy values" of fat and carbohydrate and that caloric intake is an imprecise parameter in this type of work.

The importance of the type of fat in the diet is well illustrated by the induction of hepatomas in rats fed 4-dimethylaminoazobenzene (24). Substitution of hydrogenated coconut oil for corn oil reduced the number of hepatomas obtained at six months, although the more potently carcinogenic 3'-methyl derivative did not show the effect. The fatty acids obtained from hydrogenated coconut and corn oils gave rise to similar tumor yields in experiments involving 4-dimethylaminoazobenzene. It has been suggested that the tumor-inhibitory fats enable the liver to store riboflavin more efficiently and that this led to the greater activity of detoxifying enzymes, for which riboflavin is part of a cofactor.

Beef fat (35% of diet) enhances the yield of intestinal tumors induced by azoxymethane in rats (25). The body weights of rats treated with this compound in normal and beef fat diets were similar, although those treated with beef fat diets without carcinogen were heavier. The enhancement may therefore be a direct result of the fat supplement, but it is unclear whether only beef fat is effective or if other fats could be substituted. Other aspects of experimental intestinal cancer were discussed by Reddy and co-workers (26) in a recent review.

Cycloproprenoid fatty acids may be derived from raw cotton seed oil or Sterculia foetida oil. These substances act as cocarcinogens in hepatocarcinogenesis by aflatoxin B_1 in rats. The effect on DEN carcinogenesis in rats was much less (27, 28).

Vitamin A

Vitamin A deficiency leads to squamous changes in a number of epithelial tissues, including the esophagus, bladder, and respiratory tract. The influence of this deficiency on carcinogenesis has not been studied, possibly because of the difficulty in maintaining the health of the test animals. However, there has been interest in the apparent protective effect of high levels of this vitamin since Chu and Malmgren (29) first indicated that it protected against hydrocarbon-induced tumors. Feeding 0.5% vitamin A palmitate to hamsters inhibited formation of dyskeratotic lesions, as well as carcinomas of the forestomach and small intestine, induced by 7,12-dimethylbenz(a)anthracene and B(a)P, and against esophageal dyskeratotic lesions induced by the former hydrocarbon. A considerable volume of evidence on the protective effect of dietary or topical vitamin A on skin tumor production in mice by hydrocarbons, often in combination with croton oil promotion, has been obtained (30, 31).

However, considering all tissues together, and remembering that vitamin A affects both the activation of carcinogens by the body (32) and the morphologic integrity of tissues, it is necessary to take a very guarded view of the evidence. This is perhaps most clearly indicated by studies on the effect of hypervitaminosis A on experimental lung tumors. Two studies conducted by the same highly experienced investigator have given different results—no protection, and an adverse effect (33, 34). Others have suggested a protective effect (35). Clearly more information is needed before vitamin A prophylaxis of cancer can be considered in man.

Vitamin C

Vitamin C (ascorbic acid) provides a different mechanism for the intervention of a dietary factor in carcinogenesis. In animal systems N-Nitroso compounds are known to be potent carcinogens affecting a varied range of tissues. Although no human tumors can specifically be associated with these compounds, man is known to be exposed to low levels of them from various sources. Most interestingly, they may be formed in the acid conditions of the rodent or the human stomach by reaction of the appropriate nitrogen-containing compound with nitrate. A diet rich in ascorbic acid effectively competes with the nitrogen compound for nitrite and may experimentally be shown to reduce the incidence of tumors induced by feeding the nitrogen compound with sodium nitrite. Sodium nitrite is used, among other things, as a food preservative to prevent c. botulinis contamination of food with the consequent acute, possibly fatal, poisoning. The use of ascorbate may be desirable to protect against the protective nitrite (36).

CONCLUSIONS

The examples I have discussed were drawn from a large volume of literature which was fully reviewed recently (37). These examples serve to emphasize the importance of the strict control of dietary factors as modifying agents in experimental and in human carcinogenesis. The effect of dietary factors may be at one of three phases in carcinogenesis:

1 on the way the body handles the carcinogen and either detoxifies it or converts it to an active form;
2 on the binding of the carcinogen with its critical cellular target now thought probably to be DNA; or
3 on the development of the carcinogen-affected progenitor cells into a frank, clinically observable tumor.

Possible examples of all three actions have been discussed in this paper.

In conclusion, the problem of the timing of dietary effects on the induction of spontaneous tumors will be discussed. Ross and his colleagues (38) presented outbred COBS rats with a choice of equicaloric diets containing three different levels of protein. The amount of each diet consumed was carefully monitored and it was shown that each rat, after an adjustment period, settled down to a unique standard balance of each component. Elaborate statistical analysis has so far been confined to longevity, which depends in part on tumor incidence, and it has been shown that rats consuming moderate amounts of the high protein diet in early life and moderate amounts of a carbohydrate-rich diet later in life had the greatest longevity. This is a fascinating experiment, but at this stage, difficult to interpret and more difficult to extrapolate to man. Did those rats which chose the most advantageous diet for survival do so because their disposition was directed toward this and toward long survival? These are significant questions that will have to be answered in experiments in which the elements of "choice" and "chance" are more in the hands of the investigator. This important question will then arise: Do similar findings apply to man? Are our chances of developing spontaneous or naturally occurring tumors dependent on the food presented to us in early childhood even more than on the food we consume in later life? The study of nutrition and carcinogenesis must ultimately be concerned with factors that permit the extrapolation of the results to man.

REFERENCES

1. J. A. Miller, *Cancer Res.* **30**, 559 (1970).
2. A. Tannenbaum, *Am. J. Cancer* **38**, 335 (1940).
3. A. Tannenbaum, *Arch. Pathol.* **30**, 509 (1940).
4. A. Tannenbaum, *Cancer Res.* **2**, 460 (1942).
5. C. M. McCay, M. F. Crowell, and L. A. Maynard, *J. Nutr.* **10**, 63 (1935).
6. M. H. Ross and G. Bras, *J. Nutr.* **103**, 944 (1973).
7. J. A. Saxton, G. A. Sperling, L. L. Barnes, and C. M. McCay, *Acta Unio Intern. Contra Cancrum* **6**, 423 (1950).
8. A. Tannenbaum, *Cancer Res.* **4**, 673 (1944).
9. H. Silverstone and A. Tannenbaum, *Cancer Res.* **9**, 684 (1949).
10. A. Tannenbaum and H. Silverstone, *Cancer Res.* **9**, 162 (1949).
11. H. Silverstone and A. Tannenbaum, *Cancer Res.* **11**, 442 (1951).
12. A. Tannenbaum and H. Silverstone, "Nutrition and Genesis of Tumors," *in* R. W. Raven, Ed., *Cancer,* Vol. 1, Butterworth, London (1957) p. 306.
13. M. H. Ross and G. Bras, *J. Nutr.* **103**, 944 (1972).
14. D. B. Clayson, *J. Natl. Cancer Inst.* **52**, 1685 (1974).
15. J. M. Price, *Can. Cancer Conf.* **6**, 224 (1966).
16. J. L. Radomski, E. M. Glass, and W. B. Deichmann, *Cancer Res.* **31**, 1690 (1974).
17. A. E. M. McLean and P. N. Magee, *Brit. J. Exp. Pathol.* **51**, 587 (1970).
18. D. H. Copeland and W. D. Salmon, *Am. J. Pathol.* **22**, 1059 (1946).
19. W. D. Salmon and D. H. Copeland, *Ann. N.Y. Acad. Sci.* **57**, 664 (1953).
20. P. M. Newberne, A. E. Rogers, and G. N. Wogan, *J. Nutr.* **94**, 33 (1971).
21. A. E. Rogers and P. M. Newberne, *Cancer Res.* **29**, 1965 (1969).
22. A. E. Rogers and P. M. Newberne, *Toxicol. Appl. Pharmacol.* **20**, 113 (1971).
23. A. Tannenbaum, *Cancer Res.* **2**, 468 (1942).

24. J. A. Miller and E. C. Miller, *Adv. Cancer Res.* **1**, 339 (1953).

25. N. D. Nigro, D. V. Singh, R. L. Campbell, and M. S. Pak, *J. Natl. Cancer Inst.* **54**, 439 (1975).

26. B. S. Reddy, J. Narisawa, R. Maronpot, J. H. Weisburger, and E. L. Wynder, *Cancer Res.* **35**, 3421 (1975).

27. J. E. Nixon, R. D. Sinnhuber, D. J. Lee, M. K. Landers, and J. R. Harr, *J. Natl. Cancer Inst.* **53**, 453 (1974).

28. R. O. Sinnhuber, D. J. Lee, J. H. Wales, and J. L. Ayres, *J. Natl. Cancer Inst.* **41**, 1293 (1968).

29. E. W. Chu and R. A. Malmgren, *Cancer Res.* **25**, 884 (1965).

30. W. H. Bollag, *Europ. J. Cancer* **8**, 689 (1972).

31. W. H. Bollag, *Experientia* **28**, 1219 (1972).

32. D. L. Hill, and T. W. Shih, *Cancer Res.* **34**, 564 (1974).

33. D. M. Smith, A. E. Rogers, B. J. Herndon, and D. M. Newberne, *Cancer Res.* **35**, 11 (1975).

34. D. M. Smith, A. E. Rogers, B. J. Herndon, and D. M. Newberne, *Cancer Res.* **35**, 1485 (1975).

35. U. Saffiotti, R. Montesano, A. R. Sellakumar, and S. A. Borg, *Cancer* **20**, 857 (1967).

36. S. S. Mirvish and P. Shubik, *Nature* (London) **250**, 684 (1971).

37. D. B. Clayson, *Cancer Res.* **35**, 3292 (1975).

38. M. H. Ross and E. Lustbader, *Nature* **262**, 548 (1976).

3

Dietary Factors in Hormone-Dependent Cancers

K. K. CARROLL

Department of Biochemistry, University of Western Ontario, London, Ontario Canada

Hormone-dependent cancers account for a relatively large percentage of all cancer deaths (1,2). Breast cancer, in particular, is a major cause of death among women of industrialized countries, such as the United States and Canada. Even more depressing is the apparent trend toward increased mortality from breast cancer in many countries during recent years (Fig. 1). Similar trends may be seen for other types of hormone-dependent cancer, such as prostatic cancer and ovarian cancer. Improvements in diagnosis and treatment have thus far made little impact on this serious health problem.

Preventive medicine offers a possible alternative approach to the problem, which is worthy of serious consideration. Environmental factors are thought to play an important role in carcinogenesis and may be largely responsible for geographical differences in cancer mortality, such as those seen in Fig. 1. Identification of these factors could suggest environmental changes that might be made to reduce cancer incidence and mortality.

One of our most intimate contacts with the environment is through the food we eat, and there is increasing evidence that diet can have a significant influence on carcinogenesis. This evidence comes from studies with experimental animals as well as from epidemiological data on human populations. A recent symposium, sponsored by the American Cancer Society and the National Cancer Institute, had as its theme

The author is a Medical Research Associate of the Medical Research Council of Canada.

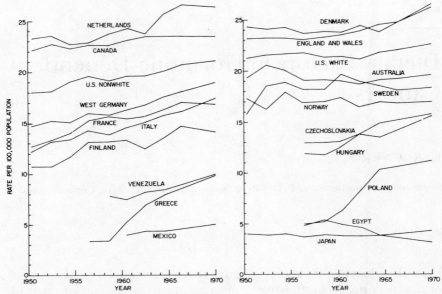

Figure 1.   Trends in age-adjusted death rates for breast cancer (female) in different countries. From data compiled by Segi et al. (1,2).

"The Role of Nutrition in the Causation of Cancer," and for a detailed discussion of the subject see (58).

This chapter is concerned with diet in relation to hormone-dependent cancers, and will deal mainly with breast cancer, since most of the experimental evidence relating diet to hormone-dependent tumors has come from studies on mammary cancer.

EFFECTS OF CALORIC INTAKE AND DIETARY FAT ON MAMMARY CARCINOGENESIS

More than 30 years ago, Tannenbaum and others showed clearly that caloric restriction inhibits development of mammary tumors in mice and rats. These experiments have been discussed in detail in reviews by Tannenbaum (3,4) and by Tannenbaum and Silverstone (5,6) and were also summarized at the symposium referred to above (7,8). Rather severe restriction to about one-half to two-thirds of the normal intake was used in most of these experiments. This appeared to inhibit the development of most types of tumors tested, including skin tumors, sarcomas, hepatomas, lung adenomas, pituitary adenomas, and leukemia, although some tumors were affected more than others. The inhibitory effect of dietary restriction may be due simply to lack of energy or metabolites required for tumor development, but it is also possible that other mechanisms, including alterations in endocrine function, may be involved in the inhibition of certain types of tumors.

Another observation made in these early studies on diet and tumorigenesis in mice and rats was that high fat diets favored development of mammary tumors in comparison to low fat diets (Fig. 2). A similar result was obtained in more recent experiments in our laboratory in which 7,12-dimethylbenz(a)anthracene (DMBA) was used to induce mammary tumors in rats (14). This effect of dietary fat appears to be more selective with respect to the type of tumor affected. For example, dietary fat had little effect on sarcomas produced by injection of carcinogenic hydrocarbons, whereas the yield of skin tumors produced by painting carcinogenic hydrocarbons on the skin was enhanced by feeding a high fat diet (4–6,15).

Stimulated by his finding that caloric restriction inhibits tumorigenesis in animals, Tennenbaum (16) surveyed several collections of insurance statistics and found some indication that cancer mortality increased with increasing body weight. In general, however, there has been little attempt until recently to relate the findings in animals to cancer incidence and mortality in human populations. Perhaps it was for this reason that interest in the effects of diet on carcinogenesis declined, and for a number of years relatively few papers were published on the subject.

The current revival of interest in the role of nutrition in carcinogenesis stems largely from analysis of epidemiological data on cancer incidence in human populations collected over the past 25 years. The incidence of different types of cancer (17) and the associated mortality (1,2) have been found to vary widely in different countries of the world. These data, together with information on migrating populations (18,19), have led to the conclusion that environmental factors are largely responsible for the observed differences (20,21). There are also increasing indications that diet may play a role in human carcinogenesis (22), including the genesis of tumors which show hormone dependency (23).

Our own studies on the enhancement of DMBA-induced mammary tumors in rats by dietary fat led us to consider the possible role of dietary fat in the development of breast cancer in humans. Examination of the epidemiological data showed a strong positive correlation between dietary fat intake and mortality from breast cancer in different countries (15,24). This is illustrated in Fig. 3, which is based on the most recent data of Segi and co-workers (2). This relationship between fat consump-

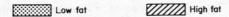

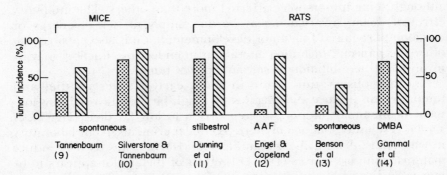

Figure 2. Effects of dietary fat on incidence of spontaneous and induced mammary tumors in mice and rats. Details of experimental procedures may be found in the original publications (9–14). AAF = 2-acetylaminofluorene; DMBA = 7,12-dimethylbenz(*a*) anthracene.

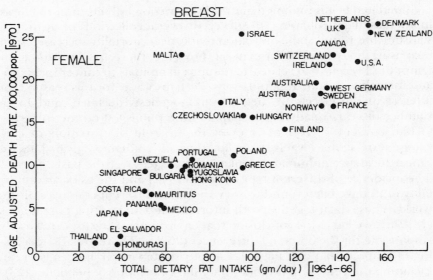

Figure 3. Correlation between per capita consumption of dietary fat (25) and age-adjusted mortality from breast cancer in different countries (2). Mortality for the United States was estimated from values given for U.S. white and U.S. nonwhite, and that for the United Kingdom from values given for England and Wales, Scotland, and Northern Ireland. Although not specified in the latest compilation, earlier data on the death rate from breast cancer in Israel was based on the Jewish population only, and this may account for its failure to conform to the correlation with fat intake. The data from Malta should probably be investigated more thoroughly to see whether there is a rational explanation for its failure to conform.

28

tion and human breast cancer mortality was also noted independently by Lea (26,27) and by Wynder (28,29).

Although one must be cautious in the interpretation of epidemiological data, the existence of a positive correlation encouraged us to pursue our studies with the animal model in order to learn more about the nature of the effect of dietary fat and the possible mechanisms by which it might influence mammary carcinogenesis in rats. In our original studies (14) corn oil was found to increase the tumor yield, whereas coconut oil had little or no effect. This suggested that the type of fat as well as the amount was important, and further confirmation was provided by experiments in which a variety of different fats and oils were fed at the level of 20% by weight of the diet (30). The number of animals that developed tumors was nearly always greater in the high fat groups than in the low fat controls, but in general, the groups of rats fed unsaturated fats were found to develop more mammary tumors following treatment with DMBA than groups fed saturated fats (Table 1). This difference was due primarily to an increase in the number of tumors per tumor-bearing rat in the groups fed unsaturated fats.

Among the unsaturated fats tested, only rapeseed oil gave a low tumor yield and it was originally suggested that this might be due to its high content of the long chain monounsaturated fatty acid, erucic acid (30). However, when this experiment was repeated, the results obtained with a diet containing 20% of high erucic rapeseed oil were comparable to those obtained with a diet containing 20% olive oil (Table 2). An even higher tumor yield was obtained with low erucic rapeseed oil, which is similar to olive oil in overall fatty acid composition. Rats on a diet containing 5% olive oil developed fewer tumors, as expected from earlier studies with low fat diets.

These data illustrate one of the difficulties with this type of experiment. Because of the variability in results from one experiment to another, it is difficult to establish the relative effectiveness of different dietary fats. Although unsaturated fats seem to give a greater enhancement of mammary tumor yields than saturated fats, it is not certain whether this difference is related to their content of essential fatty acids. For example, corn oil and soybean oil contain much more linoleic acid than olive oil, but seem to give no greater enhancement of tumor yield. Furthermore, Dayton and Hashimoto (31), using the DMBA rat mammary tumor model, have recently reported that safflower oil with normal high linoleic content was no more effective in stimulating tumorigenesis than a high oleic oil produced by a safflower mutant. It is possible, however, that increased ingestion of essential fatty acids may have an effect at lower levels of intake, and there may be a threshold above which further increases make little difference to the tumor yield.

Table 1   Effects of Different Dietary Fats and Oils on Incidence and Yield of Mammary Tumors in Rats given DMBA [a]

Dietary Fat	Av. Final Rat Body Wt. (g)	Number of Rats[b] with Tumors	Av. Number of Tumors/ Tumor- bearing Rat	Number of Tumors[c]	
				Palpable	Total
Unsaturated fats					
20% Sunflowerseed oil	248	26	4.8	88	130
20% Cottonseed oil	258	28	4.5	90	127
20% Olive oil	241	26	4.5	90	117
20% Corn oil	246	27	4.0	79	110
20% Soybean oil	252	30	3.4	77	103
20% Rapeseed oil	238	23	2.0	47	69
Saturated fats					
20% Lard	243	28	3.4	82	97
20% Butter	252	26	3.3	60	88
20% Coconut oil	247	29	2.5	55	73
20% Tallow	240	24	3.0	55	72
Low fat controls					
5% Corn oil	239	23	3.0	51	70
0.5% Corn oil	239	21	3.5	52	75

[a] Data from Carroll and Khor (30).
[b] Each group consisted of 30 female Sprague-Dawley rats.
[c] Most of the tumors were adenocarcinomas, with a few adenomas and fibro-adenomas. The total number includes nonpalpable tumors found when the rats were autopsied four months after being given the DMBA.

With respect to human populations, it can be seen from Fig. 4 that breast cancer mortality is positively correlated with animal fat intake, but not with intake of vegetal fat. Since vegetal fat tends to be more unsaturated than animal fat, this gives no indication of an association between breast cancer mortality and dietary essential fatty acids, although the picture may be complicated by the practice of hydrogenating dietary fats. The daily intake of linoleic acid by Americans is reported to be similar to that of Japanese, although the proportion relative to other fatty acids is lower (32). The proportion of linoleic acid in adipose tissue fatty acids was found to be only 10.2% in Americans compared to 16.5%

Table 2   Effects of Dietary Rapeseed Oil and Olive Oil on Incidence and Yield of Mammary Tumors in Rats given DMBA [a]

Dietary Fat[b]	Av. Final Rat Body Wt. (g)	Number of Rats[c] with Tumors	Av. Number of Tumors/ Tumor-bearing Rat	Number of Tumors	
				Palpable	Total
20% Rapeseed oil					
Low erucic acid	240	28	4.4	104	124
High erucic acid	234	25	4.0	78	100
20% Olive oil	246	27	3.9	83	107
5% Olive oil	233	26	3.3	66	85

[a] Results expressed as in Table 1.
[b] The samples of rapeseed oil were kindly donated by Proctor and Gamble, Ltd., Hamilton, Ontario, and were either low (2.3%) or high (35%) in erucic acid, as determined by gas-liquid chromatography. The olive oil was obtained from a local supermarket. The formulation of the diets and the experimental procedures were as described previously (30).
[c] Female Sprague-Dawley rats were used for these experiments. Each of the groups fed rapeseed oil comprised 29 rats, and those fed olive oil comprised 30 rats each.

in Japanese (32), whereas mortality from breast cancer is much higher in the United States than in Japan (Fig. 4).

The distribution and metabolism of linoleic acid and other essential fatty acids in the body may be influenced by a variety of factors. For example, peroxidation of polyunsaturated fatty acids is inhibited by vitamin E (33). Harman (34) reported that α-tocopherol was effective in reducing the incidence of mammary tumors in rats treated with DMBA and fed a diet containing 20% corn oil, but Dayton and Hashimoto (31) found that addition of tocopherol made no difference in their experiments with safflower oil.

DIETARY FAT AS A COCARCINOGEN

The mechanism by which dietary fat enhances mammary tumorigenesis in animals is of considerable theoretical interest and may have practical implications for human breast cancer as well. Our original experiments were based on the idea that dietary fat might alter the distribution or metabolism of the DMBA used to induce mammary tumors. Car-

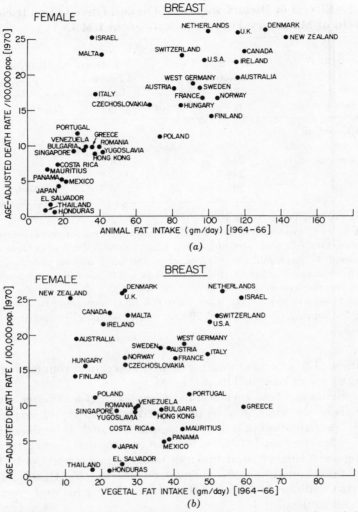

Figure 4. Correlation between per capita consumption of (*a*) animal fat and (*b*) vegetal fat, and age-adjusted mortality from breast cancer in different countries. Sources of data as for Fig. 3.

cinogenic hydrocarbons, being lipid-soluble, have a tendency to accumulate and persist in adipose tissue, and Dao and co-workers (35,36) had suggested that accumulation of these compounds in the adipose tissue of the mammary gland might account for their specificity in producing mammary cancer. However, experiments carried out in our laboratory to investigate effects of dietary fat on the accumulation and persistence of DMBA in mammary tissue gave somewhat inconclusive results (37). Furthermore, it was subsequently found that mammary tumor yields could still be increased by placing rats on a high fat diet one or two weeks after giving the DMBA (15), by which time most of the carcinogen had disappeared from the tissue (37). It should also be noted that the stimulatory effect of dietary fat has been observed with spontaneous tumors as well as with tumors induced by various carcinogenic agents (Fig. 2). It therefore seems unlikely that dietary fat exerts its effect by influencing the initial carcinogenic stimulus.

The idea that tumor development proceeds in stages (Fig. 5) was derived originally from experiments with skin tumors (38,39), but the concept is probably applicable to other kinds of tumors as well (40). On the basis of this hypothesis, dietary fat may be considered to act as a cocarcinogenic agent (41), whose effect is exerted primarily at the pre-neoplastic stage of tumor development (Fig. 5).

In the case of hormone-dependent tumors, this stage of development is greatly influenced by the hormonal environment (42,43). Some pre-liminary experiments were therefore carried out in our laboratory to investigate the effects of dietary fat on the distribution and metabolism of labeled estrogen (15), and the role of hormones in the development of mammary tumors induced by DMBA has been investigated more thoroughly by Chan and Cohen (44). Their studies led to the conclusion that dietary fat promotes mammary tumor development by increasing the concentration of circulating prolactin relative to that of estrogen. Hence it would be of interest to obtain more data on the ratio of circulat-ing prolactin to estrogen in different human populations, to see whether this ratio can be correlated with fat intake and breast cancer incidence. MacMahon and co-workers (45–47) have provided evidence of differences in urinary estrogen profiles between Asian and North American women, and have suggested that the lower ratio of estriol to estrone and estradiol in North American women may be a factor in their greater susceptibility to breast cancer.

Besides altering the hormonal environment, there are a number of other ways in which dietary fat might influence mammary tumorigenesis. Some of the possibilities have been discussed in a recent

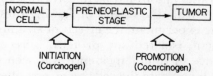

Figure 5.   Stages of tumor development.

review by Hopkins and West (48). These include effects on the structure and function of membranes, on immunocompetence, and on DNA repair potential. It is known that dietary fat can influence the fatty acid composition of tissue lipids (49), and in our intial studies on mammary cancer induced by DMBA, the fatty acid composition of rat mammary tissue was found to be markedly altered by feeding coconut oil or corn oil (14). Various properties of membranes are influenced by the fatty acid composition of membrane lipids (50), and it seems possible that alterations in membrane properties could influence susceptibility to neoplastic changes. Immunological responses to antigens associated with tumor cells may play an important role in preventing tumor development (51). There is some evidence that immunocompetence can be influenced by dietary fats (48), and this provides another possible mechanism by which dietary fat might influence tumorigenesis.

EFFECTS OF NONLIPID DIETARY CONSTITUENTS ON MAMMARY CARCINOGENESIS

In experiments with animals, the effect on mammary carcinogenesis of altering various nonlipid constituents of the diet has also been investigated (4,5,8). In general, the results have been less clear-cut than those obtained by altering the fat content of the diet. There is some evidence that restriction of dietary protein can inhibit tumorigenesis, but this effect may be related to poor weight gain associated with amino acid deficiencies. Studies have also been carried out to investigate effects of dietary vitamins and minerals, but again there has been little evidence that variations within the range compatible with good growth have much effect on tumorigenesis.

In our experiments with DMBA-treated rats, animals on commercial feed have generally developed fewer mammary tumors than those on semipurified diets, even when both diets contain about the same level of dietary fat (Table 3). Furthermore, examination of the epidemiological data on human populations has shown positive correlations between breast cancer mortality and the intake of certain nonlipid components such as animal protein and simple sugars (23,52), whereas no such correlations are seen with intakes of vegetal protein or complex carbohydrate (Figs. 6,7). These observations led us to carry out studies with DMBA-treated rats to investigate the effects of varying these nonlipid dietary constituents. In one experiment, the effects of an animal protein, casein, and a plant protein, isolated soy protein, were compared, but no significant difference in tumor incidence was seen (8). Other experiments designed to investigate the relative effects of sugars and starches

Table 3   Comparison of Incidence and Yield of Mammary Tumors in Rats Maintained on Semipurified or Commercial Diets following Treatment with DMBA [a]

Diet [b]	Av. Final Rat Body Wt. (g)	Number of Rats [c] with Tumors	Av. Number of Tumors/ Tumor-bearing Rat	Number of Tumors	
				Palpable	Total
Experiment 1					
Semipurified	239	26	2.5	52	65
Commercial	240	15	1.7	21	26
Experiment 2					
Semipurified	243	22	3.1	52	67
Commercial	245	25	1.7	26	46

[a] Results expressed as in Table 1.

[b] The semipurified diet was the same as the 5% corn oil diet in Table 1. The commercial diet was Master Fox Breeder Starter Ration (Master Feeds, Toronto, Ont.). In experiment 1, both groups were maintained on commercial diet until one week after the DMBA was given. In experiment 2, both groups were fed the semipurified diet from weaning until 50 days of age, then given commercial diet for 2 days before and 1 day after administration of DMBA as in earlier studies (30). One group was then transferred to semipurified diet while the other remained on commercial diet.

[c] Female Sprague-Dawley rats were used for these experiments. There were 29 rats in the group on commercial diet in experiment 2 and 30 rats in the other groups.

on mammary tumor incidence are in progress. Preliminary results have given some indication of higher tumor incidence associated with diets containing sugars, but this finding requires confirmation with larger numbers of animals.

Commercial feed contains considerably more dietary fiber than the semipurified diets used for our experiments, and this may be a reason for the lower tumor incidence in DMBA-treated rats on commercial feed. Low intake of dietary fiber is currently being blamed for a variety of human ills, but Drasar and Irving (52) were unable to find any correlation between dietary fiber and breast cancer in human populations. The role of dietary fiber is discussed more thoroughly by Kritchevsky (53).

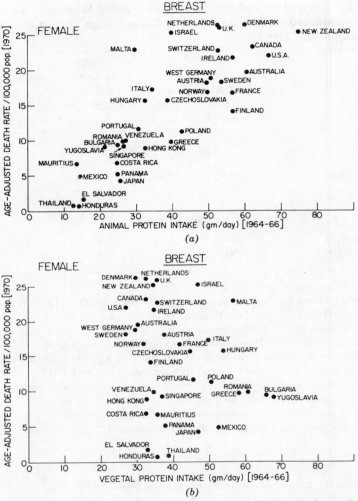

Figure 6.   Correlation between per capita consumption of (*a*) animal protein and (*b*) vegetal protein, and age-adjusted mortality from breast cancer in different countries. Sources of data as for Fig. 3.

DIET IN RELATION TO OTHER TYPES OF CANCER

The discussion up to this point has been concerned almost entirely with breast cancer, but possible effects of diet on other types of cancer will now be considered briefly, with particular reference to those that may show hormone dependency. The geographical distribution of prostatic cancer is similar to that of breast cancer (54), and it is therefore not

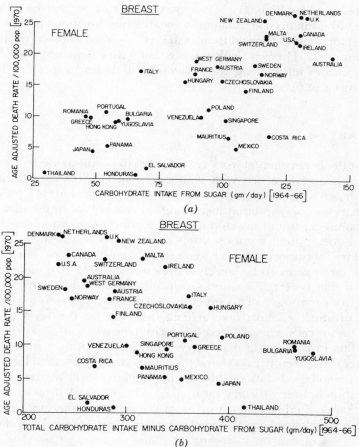

Figure 7. Correlation between per capita consumption of (*a*) sugar and (*b*) total carbohydrate less sugar, and age-adjusted mortality from breast cancer in different countries. Sources of data as for Fig. 3.

surprising to find that prostatic cancer also shows a strong positive correlation with dietary fat intake (15). In addition, the epidemiological data on human populations show positive correlations between dietary fat intake and mortality from cancer at a number of other sites in the body. These include intestinal cancer, leukemia, and cancers of the ovary, skin, and pancreas (15). Most of these would probably not be classified as hormone dependent, but it is always possible that their development may be influenced by the hormonal environment. Experimental models of intestinal cancer exist and it has been shown that yields of such tumors can be enhanced by feeding high fat diets (55). This subject is discussed in more detail by Wynder (56). A particular instance in which the diet appears to influence carcinogenesis by affecting hormone production is the development of thyroid tumors in rats subjected to prolonged iodine deficiency (57). There is also evidence that iodine deficiency may be one of the factors influencing the incidence of thyroid cancer in human populations (4,6).

SUMMARY

Most of the experimental work relating diet to hormone-dependent cancers has been concerned with mammary cancer. Studies with animals have shown that restricting caloric intake inhibits development of mammary tumors, and that increasing the level of fat in the diet stimulates mammary tumor development. The effect of caloric restriction is a general one, influencing most kinds of tumors, whereas the stimulation by dietary fat is more selective for certain types of tumors. The effect of dietary fat appears to be largely independent of caloric intake and the high fat diet is effective when given only after animals have been exposed to a carcinogen. This suggests that dietary fat acts as a promoting agent, producing a more favorable environment for the development of latent tumor cells. Unsaturated fats seem to be more effective than saturated fats in promoting mammary tumorigenesis, but it is not certain whether this difference is related to their content of essential fatty acids.

Epidemiological data on human populations show a strong positive correlation between dietary fat intake and age-adjusted mortality from breast cancer in different countries of the world. Similar, but somewhat weaker, correlations have been observed between fat intake and certain other types of cancer, including prostatic cancer and ovarian cancer. Breast cancer mortality is also positively correlated with total caloric intake, and with intakes of animal protein and simple sugars. These epidemiological data provide clues to the possible influence of different dietary components on carcinogenesis, which are being explored with the use of animal models.

ACKNOWLEDGMENTS

The contributions of Hun-Teik Khor, Susan K. Hoehn, and Reinhold Rasmussen to previously unpublished work described in this review are gratefully acknowledged. This work was supported by the Medical Research Council of Canada and the National Cancer Institute of Canada.

REFERENCES

1. M. Segi and M. Kurihara, in collaboration with T. Matsuyama, M. Ito, Y. Nagano, and K. Yamamoto, *Cancer Mortality for Selected Sites in 24Countries.* No. 6 (1966–1967) Japan Cancer Society, Nagoya, Japan, 1972.

2. M. Segi, in collaboration with K. Matsuo, K. Tomatsu, M. Tamaru, and A. Kita, *Age-adjusted Death Rates for Cancer for Selected Sites (A-Classification) in 43 Countries in 1970,* Segi Institute of Cancer Epidemiology, Nagoya, Japan, 1975.

3. A. Tannenbaum, in F. R. Moulton, Ed., *Approaches to Tumor Chemotherapy,* American Association for the Advancement of Science, Washington (1947), p. 96.

4. A. Tannenbaum, *in* F. Homburger, Ed., *The Physiopathology of Cancer,* 2nd ed., Hoeber-Harper, New York (1959), p. 517.

5. A. Tannenbaum and H. Silverstone, *in* J. P. Greenstein and A. Haddow, Eds., *Advances in Cancer Research,* Vol. 1, Academic Press, New York (1953), p. 451.

6. A. Tannenbaum and H. Silverstone, *in* R. W. Raven, Ed., *Cancer,* Vol. 1, Butterworth, London (1957), p. 306.

7. D. B. Clayson, *Cancer Res.,* **35**, 3292 (1975).

8. K. K. Carroll, *Cancer Res.,* **35**, 3374 (1975).

9. A. Tannenbaum, *Cancer Res.,* **2**, 468 (1942).

10. H. Silverstone and A. Tannenbaum, *Cancer Res.,* **10**, 448 (1950).

11. W. F. Dunning, M. R. Curtis, and M. E. Maun, *Cancer Res.,* **9**, 354 (1949).

12. R. W. Engel and D. H. Copeland, *Cancer Res.,* **11**, 180 (1951).

13. J. Benson, M. Lev, and C. G. Grand, *Cancer Res.,* **16**, 135 (1956).

14. E. B. Gammal, K. K. Carroll, and E. R. Plunkett, *Cancer Res.,* **27**,1737 (1967).

15. K. K. Carroll and H. T. Khor, *in* K. K. Carroll, Ed., *Progress in Biochemical Pharmacology,* Vol. 10, *Lipids and Tumors,* Karger, Basel (1975), p. 308.

16. A. Tannenbaum, *Arch. Pathol.,* **30**, 509 (1940).

17. R. Doll, C. Muir, and J. Waterhouse, Eds., *Cancer Incidence in Five Continents,* Vol. 2, Springer-Verlag, Berlin (1970).

18. J. Kmet, *J. Chronic Dis.,* **23**, 305 (1970).

19. W. Haenszel, *in* J. F. Fraumeni, Jr., Ed., *Persons at High Risk of Cancer, An Approach to Cancer Etiology and Control,* Academic Press, New York (1975), p. 361.

20. C. S. Muir, *in* J. F. Fraumeni, Jr., Ed., *Persons at High Risk of Cancer, An Approach to Cancer Etiology and Control,* Academic Press, New York (1975), p. 293.

21. J. Higginson, *in* J. F. Fraumeni, Jr., Ed., *Persons at High Risk of Cancer, An Approach to Cancer Etiology and Control,* Academic Press, New York (1975), p. 385.

22. E. L. Wynder, *Cancer Res.,* **35**, 3238 (1975).

23. J. W. Berg, *Cancer Res.,* **35**, 3345 (1975).

24. K. K. Carroll, E. B. Gammal, and E. R. Plunkett, *Can. Med. Assn. J.,***98**, 590 (1968).

25. *Food Balance Sheets, 1964–66 Average,* Food and Agriculture Organization of the United Nations, Rome, 1971.

26. A. J. Lea, *Lancet* **2**, 332 (1966).

27. A. J. Lea, *Ann. Roy. Coll. Surg. England,* **41**, 432 (1967).

28. E. L. Wynder, *in* A. P. M. Forrest and P. B. Kunkler, Eds., *Prognostic Factors in Breast Cancer,* Livingstone, Edinburgh and London (1968), p. 32.

29. E. L. Wynder, *Cancer* (Philadelphia), **24**, 1235 (1969).

30. K. K. Carroll and H. T. Khor, *Lipids*, **6**, 415 (1971).

31. S. Dayton and S. Hashimoto, *Abstracts IVth Intern. Sym. on Atherosclerosis*, Tokyo, Japan, 1976, Abst. F–292, p. 243.

32. W. Insull, Jr., P. D. Lang, B. P. Hsi, and S. Yoshimura, *J. Clin. Invest.* **48**, 1313 (1969).

33. A. L. Tappel, *Ann. N.Y. Acad. Sci.*, **203**, 12 (1972).

34. D. Harman, *Clin. Res.*, **17**, 125 (1969).

35. T. L. Dao, F. G. Bock, and S. Crouch, *Proc. Soc. Exp. Biol. Med.*, **102**,635 (1959).

36. F. G. Bock and T. L. Dao, *Cancer Res.*, **21**, 1024 (1961).

37. E. B. Gammal, K. K. Carroll, and E. R. Plunkett, *Cancer Res.*, **28**,384 (1968).

38. W. F. Friedewald and P. Rous, *J. Exp. Med.*, **80**, 101 (1944).

39. I. Berenblum and P. Shubik, *Brit. J. Cancer*, **1**, 383 (1947).

40. M. H. Salaman and F. J. C. Roe, *Brit. Med. Bull.* **20**, 139 (1964).

41. I. Berenblum, *in* F. Homburger, Ed., *Progress in Experimental Tumor Research*, Vol. 11, Karger, Basel (1969), p. 21.

42. J. Meites, *J. Natl. Cancer Inst.*, **48**, 1217 (1972).

43. D. Sinha, D. Cooper, and T. L. Dao, *Cancer Res.*, **33**, 411 (1973).

44. P.-C. Chan and L. A. Cohen, *Cancer Res.*, **35**, 3384 (1975).

45. P. Cole and B. MacMahon, *Lancet*, **1**, 604 (1969).

46. B. MacMahon, P. Cole, J. B. Brown, K. Aoki, T. M. Lin, R. W. Morgan, and N.-C. Woo, *Lancet*, **2**, 900 (1971).

47. B. MacMahon, P. Cole, J. B. Brown, K. Aoki, T. M. Lin, R. W. Morgan, and N.-C. Woo, *Intl. J. Cancer*, **14**, 161 (1974).

48. G. J. Hopkins and C. E. West, *Life Sci.*, **19**, 1103 (1976).

49. K. K. Carroll, *J. Am. Oil Chem. Soc.*, **42**, 516 (1965).

50. D. F. Silbert, *Ann. Rev. Biochem.*, **44**, 315 (1975).

51. F. M. Burnet, *Immunological Surveillance*, Pergamon Press, Oxford, 1970.

52. B. S. Drasar and D. Irving, *Brit. J. Cancer*, **27**, 167 (1973).

53. D. Kritchevsky, this volume.

54. E. L. Wynder, K. Mabuchi, and W. F. Whitmore, *Cancer* (Philadelphia), **28**, 344 (1971).

55. B. S. Reddy, T. Narisawa, R. Maronpot, J. H. Weisburger, and E. L.Wynder, *Cancer Res.*, **35**, 3421 (1975).

56. E. L. Wynder, this volume.

57. A. A. Axelrad and C. P. Leblond, *Cancer* (Philadelphia), **8**, 339 (1955).

58. Symposium-Nutrition in the Causation of Cancer, *Cancer Res.*, **35**,Part 2 (1975).

4

Dietary Fiber and Cancer

DAVID KRITCHEVSKY AND JON A. STORY

The Wistar Institute of Anatomy and Biology, Philadelphia, Pennsylvania

There is considerable current interest in the role of dietary fiber in the etiology of a number of diseases prevalent in the Western world. Prominent among those disease states whose prevalence is correlated with diets deficient in fiber is cancer of the large bowel. The high level of interest in the fiber hypothesis is due, in large part, to the epidemiological observations of Burkitt and his colleagues (1–3) who perceived that one factor common among diseases of the large bowel was a diet low in fiber. Drasar and Irving (4), on the other hand, correlated incidence of breast and colon cancer with a number of environmental factors and found a high positive correlation with total fat and animal protein, but practically none with dietary fiber (Table 1).

These apparently mutually exclusive observations may be explained when we consider that populations that ingest a diet high in animal products generally eat little fiber. Leveille (5) has recently reviewed the correlations between diet and incidence of cancer in Connecticut males, a group that exhibits one of the world's highest rates of colon cancer. Leveille reviewed the annual consumption of beef, meat, fish and poultry, cereals, and potatoes in this population (Table 2). Between 1935 and 1965 the incidence of colon cancer among Connecticut males had risen by 35%; consumption of beef and other meats had risen by 55 and 36%, respectively, whereas consumption of cereals had decreased by 30% and of potatoes by 26%.

Statistical analysis showed a high positive correlation with ingestion of

Supported, in part, by USPHS grants (HL–03299 and HL–05209) and a Research Career Award (HL–0734) from the National Heart, Lung and Blood Institute, and by grants-in-aid from the National Dairy Council and the National Livestock and Meat Board.

41

Table 1 Correlation between Dietary Components and Incidence of Colon Cancer[a]

Component	Correlation Coefficient
Fat	
Total	0.81
Animal	0.84
Protein	
Total	0.70
Animal	0.87
Refined sugar	0.32
Fiber and complex carbohydrate	
Total	0.02
Potatoes and starches	−0.07
Nuts	0.07
Fruit	0.22
Cereals	−0.32

[a] From Drasar and Irving (4).

Table 2 Incidence of Cancer of Large Intestine in Connecticut Males[a] as Related to United States Dietary Changes[b]

Period	Cancer 10^{5}[c]	Annual Per Capita Consumption (lbs)			
		Beef	MPF[d]	Cereal	Potatoes
1935-38	19.7	44	148	205	149
1939-42	21.2	46	165	200	140
1943-46	23.9	45	182	198	142
1947-49	25.9	51	176	170	121
1950-53	27.2	51	179	163	112
1954-57	28.9	65	192	151	111
1958-61	30.0	63	194	148	109
1962-65	30.4	68	201	144	110

[a] Age-adjusted.
[b] After Leveille (5).
[c] Incidence/100,000
[d] Meat, poultry, and fish.

beef, meat, poultry and fish, and an even higher negative correlation with consumption of cereals and potatoes (Table 3). However, all of the dietary data reveal association, not causality, and must be interpreted with caution.

Assuming that a diet high in fiber militates against colon cancer, what is the mechanism of fiber's action? Fiber in the diet shortens intestinal transit time of food and, hence, shortens residence time of potential carcinogens (6). Many types of fiber exhibit water-holding properties and, in this way, increase fecal bulk and peristaltic action (7). It has also been suggested that the intestinal flora interact with fiber to produce volatile fatty acids which exert a laxative effect (7).

Another mechanism of action involves the indirect effects of fiber on bile acid metabolism. In 1933, Wieland and Dane (8) were able, in the laboratory, to convert deoxycholic acid to methylcholanthrene, a very potent carcinogen. Deoxycholic acid itself has been found to be carcinogenic when applied to mouse skin (9). Thus these are two instances in which a bile acid is related in some fashion to carcinogenesis. Intestinal conversions of cholesterol and natural bile salts to metabolic products often found in the feces are accomplished by various intestinal microflora. Association of certain fecal steroid products with incidence of cancer and with levels of various types of bacteria yields data for further speculation.

Reddy and co-workers (10) have presented data on the spectrum of fecal steroids found in patients with colon cancer (Table 4). They showed that patients with colon cancer excreted 185% more neutral steroids and 68% more bile acids than controls. Further examination of the data shows that the ratio of cholesterol to coprostanol is increased in the patients and the ratio of primary (biosynthesized) to secondary (metabolic products) bile acids is reduced. Coprostanol and the secon-

Table 3   Correlation between Cancer of Large Intestine in Connecticut Males and Consumption of Certain Foodstuffs [a]

Consumption of	Correlation Coefficient
Beef	+ 0.905
Meat, poultry, fish	+ 0.941
Cereals	− 0.974
Potatoes	− 0.968

[a] After Leveille (5)

Table 4   Fecal Steroids (mg/g) in Patients with Colon Cancer [a]

	Patients (12)	Control (15)
Neutral		
Cholesterol (A)	13.8	3.8
Coprostanol (B)	23.0	12.6
A/B	0.60	0.30
Acidic		
Cholic acid	0.6	0.9
Chenodeoxycholic acid	0.4	0.2
Deoxycholic acid	7.2	4.2
Lithocholic acid	5.7	3.4
Other	8.1	4.4
P/S [b]	0.08	0.14

[a] After Reddy et al. (10).
[b] Primary (cholic and chenodeoxycholic)/Secondary (deoxycholic and lithocholic) bile acids.

dary bile acids are products of bacterial action. The ratio of undetermined fecal bile acids to total bile acids in controls (33.6%) and colon cancer patients (36.8%) is practically the same. Figure 1 depicts the primary and secondary bile acids.

Figure 2 shows the conversion of cholesterol to coprostanol. In Fig. 3, we see the metabolic steps which convert a bile salt to a free bile acid (via a hydrolase) and then convert the bile acid, cholic acid in this case, to a keto derivative by the action of a 7-dehydrogenase or to a secondary bile acid (deoxycholic) via a 7-dehydroxylase. These metabolic capabilities are all found in intestinal bacteria.

Hill (11) has reviewed the evidence which supports the theory that bile salts may be converted to carcinogenic hydrocarbons by bacterial action. The major reactions (Fig. 3) have been demonstrated in vivo. Other reactions which would aromatize rings A and B have been carried out in vitro using human intestinal bacteria.

Hill (11) has also reported which particular strains of bacteria exhibit the metabolic actions shown in Fig. 3. Thus no E. coli strains have hydrolase or dehydroxylase activity but 78% show 7α-dehydrogenase activity. We see that Strep. salivarius, Strep. viridans, and Lactobacillus spp. exhibit none of the enzymic activities, whereas among Strep. faecalis

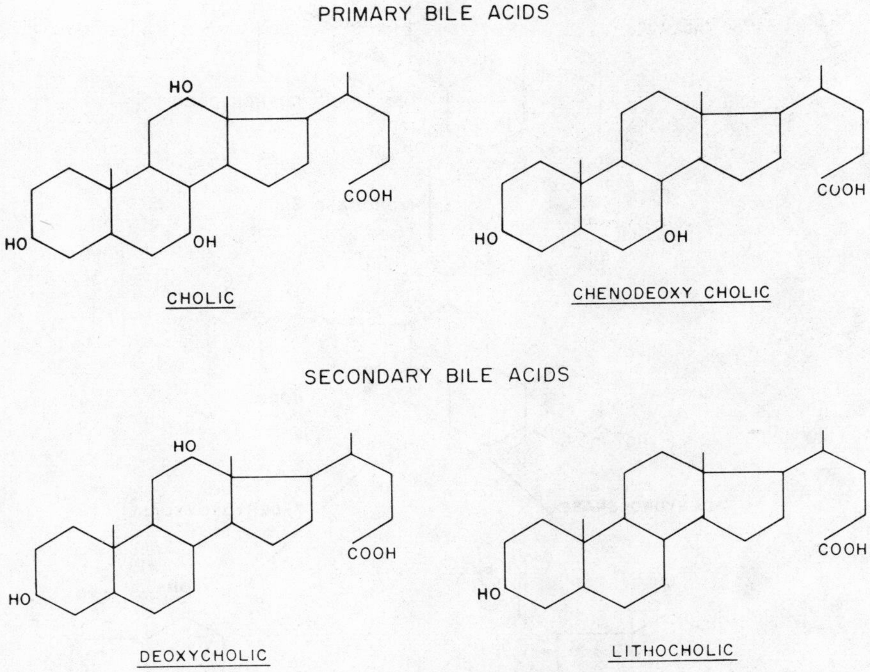
PRIMARY BILE ACIDS
HO
COOH
HO
OH
CHOLIC
COOH
HO
OH
CHENODEOXY CHOLIC
SECONDARY BILE ACIDS
HO
COOH
HO
DEOXYCHOLIC
COOH
HO
LITHOCHOLIC

Figure 1. Primary and secondary bile acids.

strains 93% contain a hydrolase, 11% a dehydroxylase, and 81% have a 7α-dehydrogenase. Among strains of Bacteroides fragilis, 82% contain a hydrolase, 44% a dehydroxylase, and 79% a 7α-dehydrogenase (Table 5).

Hill argues that dietary fiber does not influence the excretion of steroids in man and summarizes data from several experiments (Table 6) which show that addition of varying amounts of bran to the diet of a number of subjects actually resulted in a reduction of fecal steroid output.

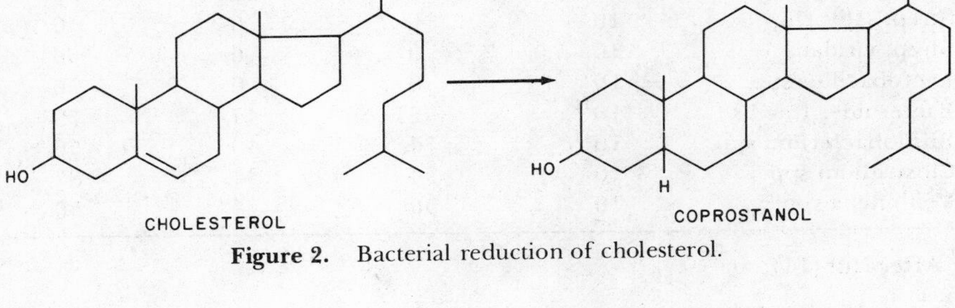
HO
CHOLESTEROL
HO
H
COPROSTANOL

Figure 2. Bacterial reduction of cholesterol.

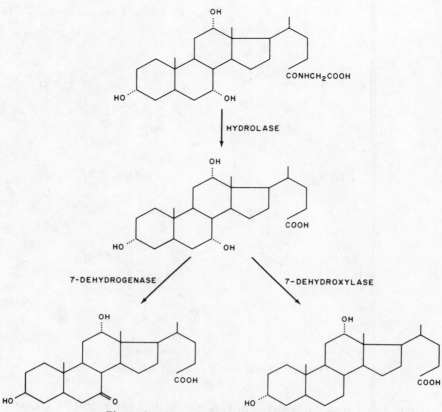

Figure 3. Bacterial action on glycocholic acid.

Table 5 Proportion of Strains of Gut Bacteria with Ability to Metabolize Bile Acids and Bile Salts [a]

Organism	No. Per Feces	Hydrolase	Percentage with Dehydroxylase	7α-dehydrogenase
E. Coli	10^8	0	1	78
Strep. faecalis	10^6	93	11	81
Strep. salivarius	10^7	0	0	81
Strep. viridans	10^7	0	0	0
Lactobacillus spp.	10^7	0	0	0
Bacteroides fragilis	10^{11}	82	44	79
Bifidobacterium spp.	10^{11}	74	40	56
Clostridium spp.	10^6	94	34	87
Veillonella spp.	10^4	50	4	50

[a] After Hill (11).

Table 6   Effect of Fiber Intake on Fecal Steroids [a]

Fiber (g/day)	No.	Wks	Percent Control Value	
			Neutral	Acidic
Bran (16)	8	3	—	61
Bran (39)	4	4	63	63
Bran (100)	4	3	56	57
Bagasse (10.5)	10	12	61	100

[a] After Hill (11).

Nigro and co-workers (12) examined the distribution of intestinal tumors experimentally induced with azoxymethane in rats fed a normal diet or one containing 2% of a bile salt-binding resin, cholestyramine. More tumors were observed on the cholestyramine-containing diet (Table 7). One explanation of this finding would be that bile acids or bile salts, even when bound, can act as cocarcinogens. It would have to be demonstrated, however, whether bile salts become metabolically inert when bound to a resin. Hill's hypothesis is that the intestinal flora, whose spectrum and activity are determined by diet, play the dominant role in colon carcinogenesis and that dietary fiber is of little consequence.

Burkitt (13) has summarized data on colon cancer incidence, gut bacteria, and fecal steroids in six populations (Table 8). In the three populations with high incidence of cancer (United States, Scotland, England) the ratio of bacteroides to streptococci is 1.7 to 1.9, the ratio of neutral to acidic steroids is under 2.0, the daily intake of fat is high, and intake of fiber is low. In the three populations with low cancer incidence (Japan, Southern India, Uganda) the ratio of bacteroides to streptococci is 1.2 to 1.3 and the ratio of neutral to acidic steroids ranges from 3 to 5. Their fiber intake was 2 to 3 times that of the more susceptible populations. In the study of Reddy and co-workers (10) (Table 4), the ratio of neutral to acidic steroids was 1.7 in the cancer patients and 1.3 in the controls.

Hill and co-workers (14) generated most of the data quoted by Burkitt (13). They obtained a virtual straight line relationship when plotting total fecal dihydroxycholanoic acids against incidence of colon cancer in six different populations. The ratio of anaerobic to aerobic bacteria present in the feces averaged 2.4 (2.1 to 2.7) in the populations with high rates of colon cancer and 1.0 (0.5 to 1.5) in those with low rates of colon cancer.

If we assume that bile acids possess cocarcinogenic properties, then their prolonged presence alone may be sufficient to enhance car-

Table 7   Distribution of Intestinal Tumors in Rats (10 group) Treated with Azoxymethane and Fed Normal Diet or One Containing 2½ Cholestyramine[a]

Site	Number of Tumors	
	Normal	Cholestyramine
Small bowel		
Proximal	36	38
Distal	5	25
Large bowel		
Proximal	20	35
Distal	9	38

[a] From Nigro et al. (12).

cinogenesis. Although bile acids have been shown to be cocarcinogenic for experimentally induced tumors (15), it remains to be proved in vivo whether the findings were due to their metabolic or to their surface active properties. In the latter case, any surface active agent would be cocarcinogenic.

If the structure of a bile acid or salt affects its role in tumorigenesis, then the extent to which it is chemically or physically bound and rendered inert may be an important factor in reducing its activity. Animal feeding studies have shown that each type of fiber has its characteristic effect on steroid excretion. Thus, alfalfa (16) can increase excretion of neutral steroids whereas pectin (17) increases excretion of bile acids.

We (18, 19) have shown that individual bile acids and salts are bound to different extents by different binding agents. As Fig. 4 shows, cellulose has a weak binding capacity and cholestyramine a strong one. Among the natural binding substances lignin exhibits the greatest binding capacity. The binding for each substrate is shown in Fig. 5. We see that lignin binds considerably more cholic acid than does alfalfa; their affinity for chenodeoxycholic acid is similar. When any specific bile acids or salts are studied, their affinity for a variety of agents should be established.

The production of colon cancer depends upon the presence of a carcinogen and, probably, the length of time of exposure. If we accept the hypothesis that bile acids are potential precursors of carcinogens and

Table 8 Cancer of the Colon and Rectum, Bacterial Flora, and Fecal Steroids [a]

				Population			
	U.S.	Scotland	England	Japan	So. India	Uganda
Incidence/100,000	41.6	51.5	38.1	13.1	14.0	3.5
Bacteria (log 10/g feces)						
Bacterioides	9.8	9.8	9.8	9.4	9.2	8.2
Streptococci	5.9	5.3	5.8	8.1	7.3	7.0
Fecal steroids (mg/g)						
Neutral	10.7 (64)[b]	10.1 (77)	10.8 (69)	4.5 (43)	1.5 (62)	1.8 (55)
Acid	6.0 (46)	6.2 (49)	6.2 (51)	0.9 (13)	0.5 (21)	0.5 (33)
N/A	1.78	1.63	1.74	5.00	3.00	3.60

[a] After Burkitt (13).
[b] % degraded.

49

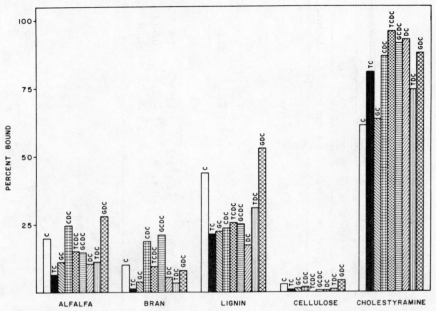

Figure 4.   Extent of binding of individual bile acids and salts by different binding agents.

we recognize that the required metabolic changes can be wrought by the intestinal bacteria, then it is important to determine which dietary factors influence bacterial proliferation. Examining the data summarized in Table 8, one may attribute the incidence of colon cancer to dietary fat, dietary animal protein, or lack of dietary fiber. Precisely how any of these components affects bacterial growth is under intense study.

If colon cancer can be related to dihydroxy bile acids (14), it should be noted that in man dietary fiber can increase the level of primary to secondary bile acids (20, 21).

It should be noted, however, that there are a few experiments relating dietary fiber to cancers other than those of the large bowel.

Wilson and De Eds (22) compared the carcinogenic action of 2-acetylaminofluorene (AAF) in rats fed diets containing 3 or 6% of crude fiber. At high levels of dietary AAF(0.125%) no difference in tumor incidence or survival time was observed, but when fed at the level of 0.062%, AAF was considerably less carcinogenic in the rats fed 6% fiber. Rats fed the 3% fiber diet survived half as long as those fed the 6% fiber diet.

Engel and Copeland (23) administered AAF to rats fed a semipurified

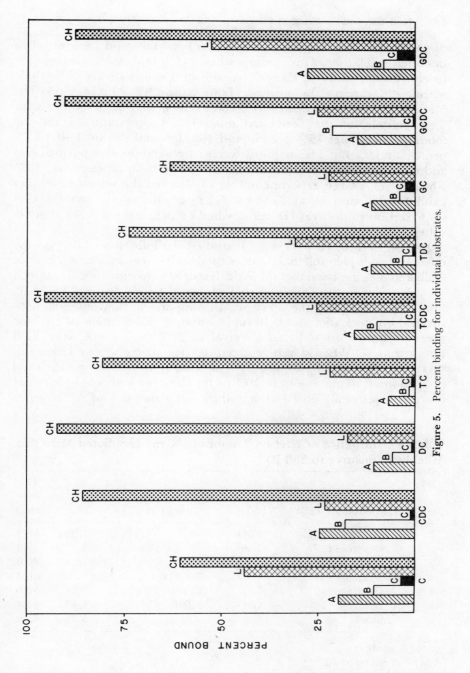

Figure 5. Percent binding for individual substrates.

diet (70% sucrose, 18% casein, 6% lard, 5% salt mix, and 1% liver oil), a modified stock diet (61.5% whole wheat, 15% lard, 9.5% sucrose, 9% casein, 4% salt mix, and 1% cod liver oil), and a stock diet (61.5% whole wheat, 12% casein, 10% meat and bone scraps, 8% skim milk powder, 5% lard, 2% alfalfa leaf meal, 1% cod liver oil, and 0.5% iodized salt). The semipurified diet contained about 18% protein and 7% fat, the modified stock diet 15% protein and 18% fat, and the stock diet 27% protein and 9% fat. The major difference between the semipurified diet and the others was that most of its sucrose had been replaced by whole wheat. Over a large experimental series, rats fed the semipurified diet exhibited 2.06 tumors/rat (97 tumors/47 rats); those on the modified diet showed 1.50 tumors/rat (18 tumors in 12 rats); and the stock diet resulted in 1.08 tumors/rat (26 tumors in 24 rats).

Ershoff and his co-workers (24) studied the influence of diet on the effects of multiple sublethal doses of total body X-ray irradiation in mice (Table 9). On the basal diet (59% dextrose, 24% casein, 10% cottonseed oil, 5% salt mix, 2% cellulose) they observed 68.3% survival and 1.02 tumors/mouse among the survivors. In comparison, they observed 65% survival on stock diet and 0.36 tumors/mouse. Substitution of lard for the cottonseed oil reduced survival to 50% and there were 2.33 tumors/mouse. When starch replaced dextrose there was no change in survival (70%) but there was a 54% increase in tumor per mouse ratio (1.57/mouse). Replacement of 10% of the dextrose with whole liver did not affect survival (66.7%) but reduced the number of tumors per

Table 9   Influence of Diet on Tumors in X-ray Irradiated Mice (Six Weekly Exposures to 200 R) [a]

Diet	Carbohydrate (1%)	Fat (10%)[b]	Other (%)	T/m[c]	(%) Survival
1	Dextrose (50)	CSO	—	1.02	68.3
2	Dextrose (59)	Lard	—	2.33	50.0
3	Starch (59)	CSO	—	1.57	70.0
4	Dextrose (49)	CSO	Liver (10)	0.70	66.7
5	Dextrose (49)	CSO	Yeast (10)	0.87	50.0
6	Dextrose (44)	CSO	Alfalfa (15)	1.75	53.3
7	Stock	—	—	0.36	65.0

[a] After Ershoff et al. (24).
[b] CSO = cottonseed oil.
[c] Tumors/mouse.

mouse to 0.70. When yeast was used to replace 10% of the dextrose, survival was only 50% but tumor/mouse ratio was 0.87.

Replacing 15% of the dextrose by alfalfa leaf meal resulted in 53.3% survival and the appearance of 1.75 tumors/mouse. The foregoing findings suggest that factors other than fiber may exert a major effect on survival and prevalence of tumors caused by X-ray irradiation. Still, if we use an arbitrary index (tumors per mouse × % survival) we find the values to be: 0.70; 1.17; 1.10; 0.47; 0.57; 0.93; 0.23 for diets 1 through 7, respectively (Table 9). The lowest value is observed in the group fed the stock diet.

The question at the moment is of the chicken-egg variety, i.e., which came first. In general, populations ingesting diets high in fiber do not eat a Western (or luxus) diet. More work is needed before we can safely ascribe enhancement or inhibition of carcinogenic potential to a specific dietary component.

REFERENCES

1. D. P. Burkitt, *J. Natl. Cancer Inst.* **47**, 913 (1971).

2. D. P. Burkitt, *Cancer* **28**, 3 (1971).

3. D. P. Burkitt, A. R. P. Walker, and N. S. Painter, *J.A.M.A.,* **229**, 1068 (1974).

4. B. S. Drasar and D. Irving, *Brit. J. Cancer* **27**, 167 (1973).

5. G. A. Leveille, *J. Animal Sci.* **41**, 723 (1975).

6. R. F. Harvey, E. W. Pomare, and K. W. Heaton, *Lancet* **1**, 1278 (1973).

7. J. H. Cummings, *Gut* **14**, 69 (1973).

8. H. Wieland, and E. Z. Dane, *Physiol. Chem.* **219**, 240 (1933).

9. G. M. Badger, J. W. Cook, C. L. Hewett, E. L. Kennaway, N. M. Kennaway, R. H. Martin, and A. M. Robinson, *Proc. Roy. Soc.* (London) Ser. B **129**, 439 (1940).

10. B. S. Reddy, A. Mastromarino, and E. L. Wynder, *Cancer Res.* **35**, 3403 (1975).

11. M. J. Hill, *in The Bile Acids, Vol. 3,* P. P. Nair and D. Kritchevsky, Eds. Plenum Press, New York (1976), in press.

12. N. D. Nigro, N. Bhadrachari, and C. Chomchai, *Dis. Colon Rectum* **16**, 438 (1973).

13. D. P. Burkitt, *in Refined Carbohydrate Foods and Disease,* D. P. Burkitt and H. C. Trowell, Eds., Academic Press, London (1975), pp. 117–133.

14. M. J. Hill, B. S. Drasar, V. C. Aries, J. S. Crowther, G. Hawksworth, and R. E. O. Williams, *Lancet* **1**, 95 (1971).

15. B. S. Reddy, T. Narisawa, R. Maronpot, J. H. Weisburger, and E. L. Wynder, *Cancer Res.* **35**, 3421 (1975).

16. D. Kritchevsky, S. A. Tepper, and J. A. Story, *Nutr. Reports Intl.* **9**, 301 (1974).

17. G. A. Leveille and H. E. Sauberlich, *J. Nutrition* **88**, 209 (1966).

18. D. Kritchevsky and J. A. Story, *J. Nutrition* **104**, 458 (1974).

19. J. A. Story and D. Kritchevsky, *J. Nutrition* **106**, 1292 (1976).

20. K. S. Mathur, M. A. Khan, and R. D. Sharma, *Brit. Med. J.* **1**, 30 (1968).
21. E. W. Pomare and K. W. Heaton, *Brit. Med. J.* **4**, 262 (1973).
22. R. H. Wilson and F. DeEds, *Arch. Ind. Hyg. Occup. Med.* **1**, 73 (1950).
23. R. W. Engel and D. H. Copeland, *Cancer Res.* **12**, 211 (1952).
24. B. H. Ershoff, G. S. Bajwa, J. B. Field, and L. A. Bavetta, *Cancer Res.* **29**, 780 (1969).

5

Diet and Cancer of the Colon

ERNST L. WYNDER AND BANDARU S. REDDY

Naylor Dana Institute for Disease Prevention, American Health Foundation, Valhalla, New York

It is surprising that the relationship between nutrition and the etiology of cancer has received relatively little attention, although marked differences in nutritional intake exist throughout the world, nutritional intake has changed considerably in all parts of the world, and these factors have indeed been correlated to variations in cancer incidence.

Nutrition may be involved in cancer causation in three ways: nutrients, food additives or contaminants may act as carcinogens, cocarcinogens or both; nutrient deficiencies may lead to biochemical abnormalities which, in turn, promote neoplastic processes; and excess intake of certain nutrients may produce metabolic abnormalities that promote neoplasms. In colon cancer, the influence of macronutrient excess that can affect the metabolism of a cell and lead to an initiation or promotion of the neoplastic process, appears to be the factor involved.

EPIDEMIOLOGIC LEADS

Epidemiological studies have contributed clues to etiological factors associated with the development of large bowel cancer (1). The major clues are the following.

1. The highest incidence rates are found in Western Europe and the Anglo-Saxon world, while the lowest incidence is found in Africa,

Work for this project was supported in part by NCI Grants NCI-CA-17613 and CA-16382 and NCI Contract NO1-CP-33305.

Asia, and South America except in Argentina and Uruguay (2,3). In general, the more economically developed a society is, the greater is its incidence of colon cancer, although Japan is an exception.

2. Among American Blacks, there are different rates in Blacks living in industrialized northern cities compared to Blacks in certain rural parts of the South (4). In Colombia, the incidence of adenomatous polyps is considerably higher in cities than in rural areas, a finding consistent with the differences in dietary habits (5).

3. There is a positive association between colon cancer and cancers of the prostate and breast, while a negative correlation exists between gastric cancer and colon cancer (6,7,8). This suggests that factors increasing the risk for cancers of the colon, breast, and prostate may reduce the risk for stomach cancer, and vice versa.

4. The sex ratio of cancer of the colon, being near unity, suggests that similar etiologic factors relating to large bowel cancer affect men and women.

5. Evidence of the importance of environmental dietary influences rather than genetic factors is documented by the higher incidence of colon cancer in American Blacks compared to African Blacks (9). The incidence is higher in the first and second generation of Japanese immigrants to Hawaii and California, compared to Japanese in Japan (10). The Seventh-Day Adventists, who consume little or no meat and concomitantly less fat than other Americans, have a relatively low rate of colon cancer (11). Of equal interest is the fact that colon cancer seems to be increasing in Japan itself, a finding consistent with the increasing Westernization of the diet (12).

6. Significant differences in colon cancer have been found between Japan and the United States, and between Puerto Rico and the United States (2,13). The fat intake is significantly lower in Japan and Puerto Rico than in the United States. There is a correlation between death rates from colon cancer and the consumption of fat in various parts of the world (Fig. 1). Although correlation does not necessarily establish causation, in the absence of such association, a causative association would be unlikely. It would appear logical to assume, even prior to metabolic studies, that diet has an influence on both fecal constituents and mucosal metabolic activity, which are likely to affect the large bowel mucosa, and that thereby malignant transformation of the cells lining the mucosa may take place.

7. Large-scale retrospective studies, in which the histories of patients with colon cancer were compared with those of control populations (14), while confirming the increased risk among patients with famil-

ial polyposis and ulcerative colitis, did not show any other factors in the medical or social history that differentiated colon cancer patients from their controls. Specifically, these studies included data on bowel movement and constipation. It would appear, therefore, that there is no evidence, at least in high risk populations, that the rate of transit time is associated with colon cancer. Also, if constipation were an important factor, women should have a higher rate of colon cancer than men because of their greater susceptibility to constipation. Neither weight, tobacco usage, nor alcohol consumption was found to relate to colon cancer incidence, nor did we find any difference in terms of socioeconomic levels of the patients.

8. Of particular interest has been the fact that the more economically developed a society is, the greater is its incidence of cancer of the colon, although not necessarily of the rectum. In low risk populations for colon cancer, right-sided colon cancer is relatively more frequent and the ratio of rectum to colon cancer is higher (15). In a recent study in Bolivia, a low risk country for the development of colon cancer, rectal carcinoma occurred more frequently than le-

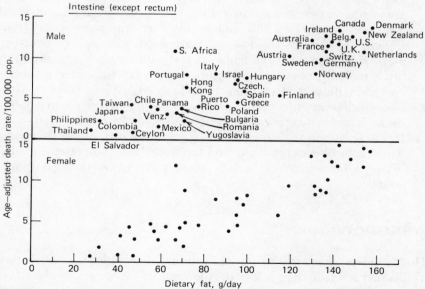

Figure 1. Correlation between the consumption of dietary fat and age-adjusted mortality from cancer of the colon.

sions of the rest of the colon (16), suggesting that the factors responsible for the development of cancer of the rectum may be different from those causing cancer of the colon.

9. Within a population, one can study the influence of socioeconomic factors. In general, it has been shown that in countries with a low rate of colon cancer, the disease is found more commonly in people of a higher economic level. However, in countries with a high rate of colon cancer, differences by socioeconomic levels are generally not observed. The absence of a socioeconomic gradient in the United States may be a reflection of the fact that the consumption of food in terms of its basic components, namely fats, proteins, and carbohydrates, tends not to differ among different population groups or regions though the source of these components obviously differs.

10. For cancer of the colon, studies in the United States have not revealed significant differences in the dietary intake of foods between cancer patients and controls (17). In Japan, on the other hand, it was shown that patients with colon cancer consumed more Westernized diets than the controls (17). Haenszel and co-workers (18) showed an association between colon cancer and dietary beef in their study of Hawaiian Japanese. In general, it must be stressed that dietary histories taken from individuals, particularly those on a Western diet, are virtually useless. Even in a dietary history of what an individual has eaten yesterday, a 25% quantitative error can be expected. This situation is obviously worse in establishing diet intakes covering many years. We must remember that if a diet history is recorded in order to study ingestion of carcinogens, we probably need information about dietary practices by individuals 20 or 30 years before. It is obvious that an individual's recollection of his earlier dietary habits is unreliable. An exception may be studies conducted in Japan or on Japanese migrants, among whom a trend toward American eating habits could be ascertained. To pinpoint which components of this Western diet might lead to this disease is obviously a difficult undertaking.

ETIOLOGIC FACTORS

These epidemiologic studies raised the question of which specific dietary factors play a role in the etiology of colon cancer. Geographic correlation between cancer frequency and national or regional consumption of select foods has been used to decide between hypotheses for testing case control studies and cohort studies.

Dietary Fat

It is generally accepted that diet, particularly high dietary fat, is a major etiologic factor, although not the sole factor, in colon cancer development. Based on Japanese data and case control, Wynder and co-workers (17) proposed that colon cancer incidence is mainly associated with high dietary fat. Haenszel and co-workers (18) noted an association between colon cancer and dietary beef. Similarly, Armstrong and Doll (6) found that the incidence and the death rate of colorectal cancer has strongly correlated with consumption of animal protein and fat. Since beef is a high fat meat, contributing about 42% of total fat calories in our population, these results supporting the relation of colorectal cancer with beef consumption are consistent with its relation to fat.

Relative to a dietary fat hypothesis it may be asked whether there is a correlation between the development of colon cancer and serum cholesterol levels. Such a correlation, which obviously exists for arteriosclerosis and myocardial infarction, in fact was not found in our retrospective studies in the United States or in Japan, nor was one found on the basis of the prospective studies carried out in Great Britain (17,19). Such a correlation probably should not have been expected since in any individual patient a correlation between the serum cholesterol level and the level of cholesterol metabolites in the feces does not necessarily exist. In view of all this, it is evident that if we are to search for the etiological factors of colon cancer in feces, descriptive epidemiology cannot advance our knowledge, and by necessity, we must rely on metabolic or biochemical epidemiology, a study in which we apply classical epidemiology techniques to metabolic parameters in man.

Dietary Animal Protein

Gregor and co-workers (20) correlated cancer mortality with food consumption and found a high correlation between animal protein consumption and colon cancer incidence. Drasar and Hill (21) have discussed a number of carcinogens and cocarcinogens that could be produced by the intestinal bacteria from amino acids and that could, therefore, be seen as intermediaries linking dietary protein and colon cancer. None of these compounds has been studied yet for colon carcinogenesis. Demographic studies indicate that the incidence of colorectal cancer in a population is related principally to consumption of meat (18) and fat (17,22). These two dietary components are closely related because a high proportion of our dietary fat is derived from meat.

Dietary Fiber

Burkitt and co-workers (23) have related the risk of large bowel cancer to the use of refined sugar and the deficiency of dietary fiber, and have further pointed out that in high risk populations the elevated consumption of refined carbohydrates and the lack of dietary fiber increase the intestinal transit time and reduce the stool bulk. It has been suggested that carcinogens produced by the action of intestinal bacteria, when held for a prolonged period in contact with colon mucosa, account for the high incidence of colon cancer. There is no support for the belief that an increased transit time results in a decreased microbial action on colonic contents.

When judged on a worldwide basis, there is no correlation between the fiber content of foods and the incidence of colon cancer (24). Studies by Haenszel and co-workers (18) indicate, in fact, a positive correlation between colon cancer and the consumption of legumes that are high in fiber content. It is unlikely, therefore, that either the deficiency of dietary fiber, transit time of the stool, or dietary excess of refined sugars is an important factor in the etiology of large bowel cancer.

Other Factors

Selikoff and co-workers (25) have presented evidence that asbestos workers have an increased risk of developing colon cancer. If this should indeed prove to be the case, it will be of interest to consider the mechanism whereby asbestos fibers increase the chances of developing large bowel cancer. This lead should be explored further, both epidemiologically and experimentally.

HYPOTHESIS ON THE ETIOLOGY OF COLON CANCER

The epidemiological findings suggest an association of large bowel cancer with high dietary fat and perhaps with a specific dietary component such as beef. Most experimental studies have supported the role of dietary fat. Wynder and co-workers (17) first proposed that the feces of high and low risk groups for large bowel cancer should be examined for biochemical and bacteriological differences, since the intestinal microflora may possibly play a role in converting an inactive precursor to an active carcinogen. The relationship between dietary fat and large bowel cancer has been explained on the basis that high dietary fat increases the concentration of bile acids and neutral steroids in the large bowel and also increases the concentration of certain bacteria of the colon, and that the gut microflora metabolize these bile acids and neutral sterols to carcinogens or cocarcinogens, or both, active in the large bowel (26). Historically, certain bile acids and neutral sterols are of interest because they show steric similarity to carcinogenic polycyclic aromatic hydrocarbons and because the human gut flora have been assumed to achieve partial aromatization of the steroid ring (27–29). It would appear unlikely that such bacteria-mediated reactions could yield polycyclic aromatic hydrocarbons. They are much more likely to give products which can be metabolized to carcinogens in the mucosa or which can act as colon tumor promoters rather than as complete carcinogens.

Although no carcinogen has yet been identified in colon carcinogenesis, based on our studies (30–33) and those of others (34–36), the following hypothesis on the etiology of colon cancer is suggested.

1. Conversion of cholesterol and $\Delta^{5,7}$-dehydrocholesterol which are normally found in colonic contents and mucosa, by electrol oxidation to reactive metabolites that are capable of interacting with a nucleophile and act as carcinogens may be an important step in colon carcinogenesis.
2. Mucosal or luminal conversion of cholesterol to its epoxide may be of etiologic significance since its further conversion product, triol, has been identified in feces.
3. Dietary fat or meat changes the concentration of fecal bile acids and cholesterol metabolites and also the metabolic activity of colon bacteria which may produce tumorigenic compounds from bile acids. These bile acids act as colon tumor promoters, but not complete carcinogens.
4. Diet also influences mucosal microsomal enzymes, which could play a role in modifying colon carcinogenesis.

EXPERIMENTAL STUDIES IN ANIMAL MODELS

Promoting Effect of Bile Acids

The effect of bile acids in colon carcinogenesis has received substantial support from animal studies. Several bile acids were found to induce sarcomas at injection site, but not carcinomas, in animal models (28). This particular evidence of oncogenic effect, in fact, is not relevant to the question of whether select bile acid or cholesterol metabolites can induce carcinomas in the colon. Nigro and co-workers (37) and Chomchai and co-workers (38) observed that an increase of bile salts in the colon of rats, induced either by feeding cholestyramine or by surgically diverting bile to the middle of the small intestine, enhanced colon tumor formation. Narisawa and co-workers (30) have reported that both taurodeoxycholic acid and lithocholic acid act as colon tumor promoters in conventional rats, while Reddy and co-workers (31,39) have shown that deoxycholic acid, lithocholic acid, cholic acid, and chenodeoxycholic acid also do this in germ-free and conventional rats (Table 1).

Modifying Effect of Dietary Fat in Colon Carcinogenesis

The possible role of dietary fat in the induction of large bowel cancer in man has received some support from experimental studies. Rats fed diets containing either 20% lard or 20% corn oil had a higher incidence

Table 1   Promoting Effect of Bile Acids of Colorectal Tumor Induction by Intrarectal (i.r.) N-methyl-N'-nitro-N-nitrosoguanidine (MNNG) in Germfree and Conventional Fischer Rats

Treatment	Animals with Tumors %	Animals with Tumors No.	Tumor Classification Total	Tumor Classification Adenocarcinoma	Tumor Classification Adenoma
Conventional[a]					
LC (32)	0	0	0	0	0
TDC (32)	0	0	0	0	0
MNNG (32)	25	8	10	5	5
MNNG and LC (29)	52	15	30	8	22
MNNG and TDC (29)	62	18	28	4	24
Germfree[b]					
DC (10)	0	0	0	0	0
MNNG (16)	89	14	38	7	31
MNNG and DC (22)	82	18	75	28	47

[a] MNNG group was given single dose of 4 mg i.r. MNNG; LC (lithocholic acid) or TDC (taurodeoxycholic acid) group received 1 mg bile acid i.r. 5 times/week for 13 months; the MNNG and LC or MNNG and TDC groups were given i.r. MNNG and bile acid, as above (30).
[b] MNNG group was given MNNG i.r., 2 mg/rat, twice weekly for four weeks; DC group received deoxycholate i.r., 20 mg/rat, three times weekly for 50 weeks; MNNG and DC group received MNNG and bile acid as above (31).

of DMH-induced colon tumors than rats fed diets with 5% lard or 5% corn oil (40). Recent data by Reddy and co-workers (41) also indicate that a high beef, high fat diet or a high soybean protein, high corn oil diet led to more DMH-induced colon tumors in rats than control diets. Fecal excretion of bile acids and cholesterol metabolites was higher in rats fed high fat diets than in those fed low fat diets (42).

Other Dietary Factors

Micronutrients such as vitamin A and lipotropes have been shown to influence colon carcinogenesis in experimental animals. There was a positive association between the incidence of colon cancer, marginal vitamin A deficiency, and decreased serum and tissue levels of vitamin A in rats fed aflatoxin B_1 (43). Chronic dietary deficiency of vitamin A slightly increased the DMH-induced colon tumors in rats (44). However, intrarectal administration of the direct acting MNNG induced fewer colon tumors in vitamin A-deficient rats compared to vitamin A-supplemented animals (45). These contrasting findings require additional exploration of underlying mechanisms.

The possible role of dietary lipotropes in colon cancer has been studied by Rogers and Newberne (44), who showed that rats fed a diet deficient in lipotrope factors were more sensitive to DMH-induced colonic tumors. Since this diet was also high in fat, the observed effects could be also due to this, or to the deficiency in lipotropic factors, or both.

METABOLIC STUDIES IN MAN

Several laboratories have carried out studies to determine whether changes in the diet would alter the activity of fecal bacteria and the concentration of fecal bile acids and neutral sterols, and also whether differences in fecal constituents occur in patients with colon cancer, or patients with other large bowel diseases who constitute a high risk for the development of colon cancer.

Fecal Constituents of Populations with Diverse Dietary Habits

In relation to fat, Hill and co-workers (35) observed a correlation between the death rate due to colon cancer in various populations with diverse dietary habits and fecal excretion of bile acids and neutral sterols and fecal bacterial flora. Reddy and Wynder (32) found that the populations on a high fat, mixed Western diet, among whom the rate of colon cancer is high, excreted high amounts of bile acids and cholesterol metabolites, and also showed higher fecal bacterial β-glucuronidase activity compared to people with a comparatively low rate of colon cancer (Table 2). Since many exogenous and endogenous substances, including important tumorigenic metabolites, are excreted via bile as glucuronide conjugates, the data imply that the colonic bacteria of high risk groups are more active in hydrolyzing the conjugates than those of low risk groups. In another study, comparing a high meat, high fat diet with no meat, low fat diet, showed that the former resulted in an elevated level of fecal bile acids and cholesterol metabolites and fecal bacterial β-glucuronidase activity (33,46) (Table 3). Studies in which the protein content was altered without changing the fat content of the diet revealed no great change in the fecal bacterial flora. This suggests that the fat in the meat controls the effect on fecal constituents (47).

Table 2   Daily Fecal Excretion of Neutral Sterols and Bile Acids and Fecal Bacterial β-glucuronidase Activity in Different Populations[a]

	Americans on a Mixed Western Diet (17)	American Vege- tarians (12)	American Seventh- Day Adventists (11)	Japanese (17)	Chinese (11)
Neutral sterols (mg/day)					
Cholesterol	30.3	66.5	74.0	145	74.9
Coprostanol	571	231	178	109	102
Coprostanone	217	20.0	13.6	12.4	17.9
Total	817	318	266	266	195
Bile acids (mg/day)					
Cholic acid	8.48	6.84	1.14	5.27	2.98
Deoxycholic acid	106	32.3	24.7	40.0	22.1
Lithocholic acid	81.1	23.4	15.0	22.8	20.0
Total bile acids	256	133	54.0	83.8	54.0
β-glucuronidase activity/day/10^{-3}	425	73	180	61	66

[a] Data from Reddy and Wynder (32).

Table 3   Effect on Non-meat Diet on Fecal Excretion of Neural Sterols and Bile Acids and on Fecal Bacterial β-glucuronidase Activity [a]

	High Fat/ High Meat Mixed Western Diet (8)	Non-meat Diet (8)
Neutral sterols (mg/g dry feces)		
Cholesterol	2.6	2.7
Coprostanol	21.1	14.2
Coprostanone	4.5	2.2
Total	28.2	19.1
Bile acids (mg/g dry feces)		
Cholic acid	0.69	1.60
Chenodeosycholic acid	0.10	0.24
Deoxycholic acid	4.37	2.60
Lithocholic acid	2.96	3.02
12-Ketolithocholic acid	0.40	0.23
3,12-Diketo-5β-cholanic acid	0.14	0.08
3-Keto-5β-cholanic acid		
3α,12α-Dihydroxy-7-keto-5 β-cholanic acid	0.07	0.07
3α-Hydroxy-7-keto-5β-cholanic acid	0.04	0.04
Other bile acids	3.82	3.23
Total bile acids	12.80	11.20
Fecal bacterial β-glucuronidase activity/mg dry feces	35.0	9.2

[a] Data from Reddy, Weisburger, and Wynder (33).

In summary, the results of experiments conducted in several laboratories indicate that high dietary fat affects the metabolic activity of the intestinal bacteria as well as levels of certain bile acids and cholesterol metabolites which can act as colon tumor promoters.

Fecal Constituents of Patients with Colon Cancer

Comparisons of fecal constituents in terms of bacteria, bile acids, and neutral sterols were carried out on patients with colon cancer. Hill and co-workers (36) found that the patients with colon cancer had increased levels of fecal bile acids and nuclear dehydrogenating Clostridia compared to controls. Reddy and co-workers (48) have also shown that the concentration of fecal bile acids and cholesterol metabolites in colon cancer patients is higher than in controls, as is fecal 7α-dehydroxylase activity (49), which could result in the liberation of possible substances proven to be tumor promoters in animal models (Table 4). Although

Table 4   Fecal Neutral Sterols and Bile Acids Excretion and Fecal 7α-dehydroxylase and Cholesterol Dehydrogenase Activity in Patients with Colon Cancer and Controls [a]

	Controls (31)	Colon Cancer Patients (31)
Neutral sterols (mg/g dry feces)		
Cholesterol	2.97	10.68
Coprostanol	12.44	17.53
Coprostanone	2.10	3.61
Cholestan-3β,5α,6β-triol	0.04	0.14
Total	17.55	31.96
Bile acids (mg/g dry feces)		
Cholic acid	0.32	0.54
Chenodeoxycholic acid	0.26	0.57
Deoxycholic acid	3.76	6.96
Lithocholic acid	3.13	6.41
Other bile acids [b]	3.38	5.19
Total	10.85	19.87
7 α-dehydroxylase activity/ 100 mg dry feces	38.3	68.0
Cholesterol dehydrogenase activity/100 mg dry feces	20.8	55.5

[a] Data from Reddy and Wynder (48) and Mastromarino, Reddy, and Wynder (49).
[b] Other bile acids include ursodeoxycholic acid, 3-keto-5β-cholanic acid, 7-keto-lithocholic acid, 12-ketolithocholic acid, 7,12-diketolithocholic acid, and other microbially modified bile acids.

species of Clostridium (not the paraputrificum group or NDC group) constituted a greater percentage of the fecal flora in patients with colon cancer, the differences observed in our studies are not significant. In the NDC group, about 35% of colon cancer patients and 20% of controls had one or more Clostridium belonging to the group.

PREVENTIVE MEASURES

From the foregoing it might well be asked what kind of preventive suggestions are in order, both in terms of individual eating habits and in terms of the food industry which controls the type of food a society has available to use and thus consumes. As present evidence suggests, the "Japanese type" diet tends to protect against colon cancer while ours tends to promote it (Fig. 2). The major differences in these diets relate to the total caloric intake, and particularly to the intake of fat and cholesterol. From the point of view of preventing atherosclerosis, a Prudent Diet has long been suggested, i.e., reducing fat intake to approximately 35% of total calories and reducing cholesterol to 300 mg/day (Fig. 3). It is quite possible that the stricter type of Prudent Diet suggested by Connor and Connor (50), i.e., fat intake accounting for only 20% of total

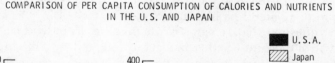

COMPARISON OF PER CAPITA CONSUMPTION OF CALORIES AND NUTRIENTS
IN THE U.S. AND JAPAN

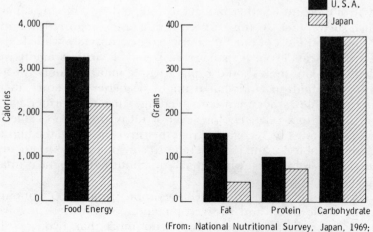

(From: National Nutritional Survey, Japan, 1969;
National Food Situation, U.S.A., 1968)

Figure 2. Nutrient consumption in the United States and Japan.

PRUDENT DIET AND PRESENT AMERICAN DIET

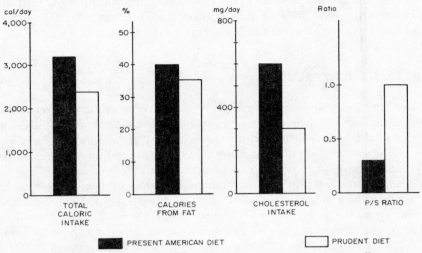

Figure 3.   Composition of Prudent Diet and present American diet.

calories and cholesterol limited to 100mg/day, would be the optimal type of diet for a sedentary population not only for prevention of coronary disease but, in our opinion, for reducing those types of cancers which seem to be related to a high fat intake.

The question that remains is whether we, as individuals, can adopt this type of diet and whether in fact our food industry has the capacity to produce such a diet. In this respect, it must be recognized that in very early childhood most of our fat calories come from milk while later they come from meat. From a managerial point of view, it might well be decided that skim milk should replace whole milk, not only for adults, but also for children, and that it might be better to return to range feeding of cattle rather than corn feeding, since the former has been shown to lead to a relatively low level of fat in the meat (Table 5). As individuals, it must be recognized that the rarer the meat, the higher the fat content (Table 5), and that we tend to consume most of our meat in the form of hamburgers, which make up about half the meat intake in the American population.

As for cholesterol, the egg contributes approximately 60% of our total intake of cholesterol, and the recommendation by those involved in coronary heart disease prevention that not more than two eggs should be consumed per week is probably a conservative one. The egg white is obviously very nutritious in the absence of the yolk. Research should be

Table 5   Fat Content of Beef as Affected by Type of Cooking and Methods of Raising Beef Cattle

	Sirloin Steak from	
Extent Cooked	Grass-fed Beef Cattle	Grain-fed Beef Cattle
	% Fat/Dry Matter	
Raw	23.7	53.8
Rare	22.0	51.7
Medium	20.5	44.6
Well done	18.2	36.1

carried out to determine to what extent the cholesterol in eggs can be reduced without affecting the taste.

Finally, it must be recognized that just as the number of fat cells appear to be determined very early in life (51), certain factors relating to fat and cholesterol metabolism may also be set quite early in life. It behooves us, therefore, to develop optimal diets, that is, diets that on the one hand make optimal growth of our bodily and intellectual functions possible while, on the other hand, not providing an excess of macronutrients which our bodies are not able to properly metabolize.

Finally, it might be asked whether a low fat, low cholesterol diet should be recommended for patients with solitary polyps. We would like to see a careful clinical study undertaken in this regard.

In summary, it is our belief that it is prudent to adopt a Prudent Diet, one lower in calories, fat, and cholesterol than the present American diet, which appears to be especially injurious to a largely sedentary population both in terms of cardio-vascular disease (the largest cause of death in our adult population) and in the development of several types of cancers, including cancer of the colon.

REFERENCES

1. E. L. Wynder, *Cancer Res.*, **35**, 3388 (1975).
2. R. Doll, *Brit. J. Cancer*, **23**, 1 (1969).
3. J. W. Berg and M. A. Howell, *Cancer*, **34**, 807 (1974).
4. W. Haenszel and E. A. Dawson, *Cancer*, **18**, 265 (1965).
5. P. Correa and G. Llanos, *J. Natl. Cancer Inst.*, **36**, 717 (1966).
6. B. Armstrong and R. Doll, *Int. J. Cancer*, **15**, 617 (1975).
7. J. W. Berg, *Cancer Res.*, **35**, 3345 (1975).

8. W. Haenszel and P. Correa, *Cancer Res.,* **35**, 3452 (1975).

9. U.I.C.C., *in* R. Doll, C. S. Muir, and J. Waterhouse, Eds., *Cancer Incidence in Five Continents,* Vol. 2, Springer Verlag, Berlin (1970).

10. W. Haenszel and M. Kurihara, *J. Natl. Cancer Inst.,* **40**, 43 (1968).

11. R. L. Phillips, *Cancer Res.,* **35**, 3513 (1975).

12. P. Correa and W. Haenszel, "Comparative International Incidence and Mortality," *in* D. Schottenfeld, Ed., *Cancer Epidemiology and Prevention,*Charles C. Thomas, Springfield (1975), p. 386.

13. I. Martinez, R. Torres, and Z. Frias, *Cancer Res.,* **35**, 3265 (1975).

14. E. L. Wynder and T. Shigematsu, *Cancer,* **20**, 1520 (1967).

15. W. W. deJong, N. E. Day, and C. S. Muir, *Intl. J. Cancer,* **10**, 463 (1972).

16. J. Rios-Dalenz, L. R. Smith, and T. F. Thompson, *Am. J. Surgery,* **129**, 654 (1975).

17. E. L. Wynder, T. Kajitani, S. Ishikawa, H. Dodo, and A. Takano, *Cancer,***23**, 1210 (1969).

18. W. Haenszel, J. W. Berg, M. Segi, M. Kurihara, and F. B. Locke, *J. Natl. Cancer Inst.,* **51**, 1765 (1973).

19. G. Rose, H. Blackburn, A. Keys, H. L. Taylor, W. B. Kannel, O. Paul, D. D.Reid, and J. Stalmer, *Lancet,* **1**, 181 (1974).

20. O. Gregor, R. Toman, and F. Prusova, *Gut,* **10**, 1031 (1969).

21. B. S. Drasar and M. J. Hill, *Human Intestinal Flora,* Academic Press, New York (1974), pp. 191–225.

22. E. L. Wynder and B. S. Reddy, *J. Natl. Cancer Inst.,* **54**, 7 (1975).

23. D. P. Burkitt, *J. Natl. Cancer Inst.,* **54**, 3 (1975).

24. B. S. Drasar and D. Irving, *Brit. J. Cancer,* **27**, 167 (1973).

25. I. J. Selikoff, E. C. Hammond, and H. Seidman, "Cancer Risk of Insulation Workers in the United States," *in* P. Bogovski, Ed., *Biological Effects of Asbestos,* I.A.R.C., Lyon (1975).

26. V. C. Aries, J. S. Crowther, B. S. Drasar, M. J. Hill, and R. E. O. Williams, *Gut,* **10**, 334 (1969).

27. M. M. Coobs, T. S. Bhatt, and C. J. Croft, *Cancer Res.,* **33**, 832 (1973).

28. A. Lacassagne, N. P. Buu-Hoi, and F. Zajdela, *Nature,* **209**, 1026 (1966).

29. M. J. Hill, *Am. J. Clin. Nutr.,* **27**, 1475 (1974).

30. T. Narisawa, N. E. Magadia, J. H. Weisburger, and E. L. Wynder, *J. Natl. Cancer Inst.,* **55**, 1093 (1974).

31. B. S. Reddy, T. Narisawa, and J. H. Weisburger, *J. Natl. Cancer Inst.,* **56**,441 (1976).

32. B. S. Reddy and E. L. Wynder, *J. Natl. Cancer Inst.,* **50**, 1437 (1973).

33. B. S. Reddy, J. H. Weisburger, and E. L. Wynder, J. Nutr., **105**, 878(1975).

34. M. Wilk and W. Taupp, *Zeitschr. Naturforsch.,* **24B**, 16 (1969).

35. M. J. Hill, B. S. Drasar, V. C. Aries, J. S. Crowther, G. M. Hawksworth, and R. E. O. Williams, *Lancet,* **1**, 95 (1971).

36. M. J. Hill, B. S. Drasar, R. E. O. Williams, T. W. Meade, A. G. Cox, J. E. P. Simpson, and B. C. Morson, Lancet, **2**, 535 (1975).

37. N. D. Nigro, N. Bhadrachari, and C. Chomchai, *Dis. Colon Rectum,* **16**,438 (1973).

38. C. C. Chomchai, N. Bhadrachari, and N. D. Nigro, *Dis. Colon Rectum,* **17**,310 (1974).

39. B. S. Reddy, unpublished results, 1976.

40. B. S. Reddy, T. Narisawa, D. Vukusich, J. H. Weisburger, and E. L. Wynder, *Proc. Soc. Exp. Biol. Med.*, **151**, 237, (1976).

41. B. S. Reddy, T. Narisawa, and J. H. Weisburger, *J. Natl. Cancer Inst.*, **57**,567 (1976).

42. B. S. Reddy, *Cancer*, **36**, 2401 (1975).

43. P. M. Newberne and A. E. Rogers, *J. Natl. Cancer Inst.*, **50**, 439 (1973).

44. A. E. Rogers and P. M. Newberne, *Cancer Res.*, **35**, 3428 (1975).

45. T. Narisawa, B. S. Reddy, C. Q. Wong, and J. H. Weisburger, *Cancer Res.*, **36**,1379 (1976).

46. B. S. Reddy, J. H. Weisburger, and E. L. Wynder, *Science*, **183**, 416(1974).

47. B. R. Maier, M. A. Flynn, G. C. Burton, P. K. Tsutakawa, and D. J. Hentges, *Am. J. Clin. Nutr.*, **27**, 1470 (1974).

48. B. S. Reddy and E. L. Wynder, *Cancer*, in press.

49. A. Mastromarino, B. S. Reddy, and E. L. Wynder, *Am. J. Clin. Nutr.*, in press.

50. W. E. Connor and S. L. Connor, *Prev. Med.*, **1**, 69 (1973).

51. C. J. Glueck, R. Tsang, W. Balistreri, and R. Fallat, *Metabolism*, **21**,1181 (1972).

PART 2

Nutrient Deficiencies

6

Cancer Cachexia

ATHANASIOS THEOLOGIDES, M.D., Ph.D.

University of Minnesota Medical School, Minneapolis, Minnesota

Cachexia, one of the hallmarks of advanced cancer, has been observed in one-third to two-thirds of patients with various cancers (1–3). It was the most frequent single cause of death in cancer prior to the introduction of aggressive radiotherapeutic and chemotherapeutic management of the disease (4,5), and its incidence may even have increased with the prolongation of survival achieved in various metastatic cancers.

The major clinicopathologic characteristics of cancer cachexia are anorexia, early satiety, increased basal metabolic rate and energy expenditure despite the reduced caloric intake, loss of body protein, fat, and other components leading to a significant weight loss, abnormalities in carbohydrate metabolism, water and electrolytic abnormalities, anemia, and marked asthenia.

Cancer cachexia is a genuine clinical syndrome that may be reversible when the total malignant growth is removed, or when complete remission of the cancer is achieved with radiotherapy or chemotherapy. For example, an uncomplicated cancer of the kidney may cause malignant cachexia that is reversed upon resection of the cancer (6). A complete chemotherapeutic remission of disseminated lymphoma may be followed by reversal of the process of an advancing cachexia.

ANOREXIA AND EARLY SATIETY

Anorexia is a common symptom in cancer that can occur as an early manifestation of the disease and disappear completely after curative

This research was supported in part by grants No. CA-08832, CA-16450, and CA-19527 from the National Cancer Institute of the United States Public Health Service, the Masonic Hospital Fund, Inc., and the Minnesota Medical Foundation.

resection. It may also appear as the malignant neoplasm grows and spreads, and it is always present as a part of the cachexia syndrome. Psychological, emotional, and therapeutic factors, and complications of the disease and the treatment may initiate or worsen the anorexia, but as the disease progresses, it is usually the cancer itself that is the main cause of the anorexia (7).

The pathogenesis of anorexia in cancer remains unexplained. Actually, even major phases of the normal physiology of hunger and satiety continue to remain conjectural.

In the brain, there is a regulatory system with the hypothalamus playing a major facilitatory and inhibitory role for hunger and satiety, and with neocortical and limbic systems participating in the regulation (8). The ventromedial nuclei of the hypothalamus are the "satiety" centers and the lateral nuclei are the "feeding" centers; higher regions exert modifying influences. At present, there is no evidence that a malfunction of the brain centers is the cause of the anorexia of cancer.

The signals and messages that could stimulate or suppress feeding and satiety centers in the brain remain speculative for the most part. The proposed theories suggest neural, physical, and chemical signals and messages working on peripheral and central receptors.

The alimentary tract regulation theory states that sensations from the oropharyngeal regions, the stomach, and the intestine play a regulatory part by metering the quantity of food eaten on a meal-to-meal basis (9–12). The regulation by osmoreceptors indicates that the water concentration or shift of water from intracellular to extracellular compartments generates satiety signals transmitted to the brain (13–14). The thermostatic hypothesis proposes that the heat released during the assimilation of food, the "specific dynamic action" of food, is the force that regulates the food intake on a day-to-day basis (15–16). The glucostatic regulation emphasizes that the rate of glucose utilization, the "effective blood sugar," provides the link between the supply of nutrients and the hypothalamus (17–19). The lipostatic hypothesis considers a circulating, humoral factor to be in dynamic equilibrium with the total adipose tissue in the body. This factor supposedly is the signal for the brain centers whose primary long-term regulation is the stabilization of fat stores (20). In amino acid regulation, the concentration and the pattern of amino acids in the blood and extracellular fluid are considered to be important signals for regulating food intake (21,22). In hormonal regulation, insulin, growth hormone, glucagon, enterogastrone, and cholecystokinin have been proposed as factors causing hunger or satiety and as playing an important role in the short-term regulation of food intake (23–30). In a metabolic theory, the regulation of the work of the hypothalamic centers is linked to a phase of the intermediary metabolism and, most specifically, to the tricarboxylic acid cycle (31).

All of these theories, however, leave major questions on the physiology and pathophysiology of hunger and satiety unanswered, and none of them can explain the pathogenesis of anorexia in cancer (32). It appears that a complex mechanism normally regulates food intake, with several feeding and satiety signals and messages contributing to the regulation through a peripheral and central effect. The satiety signals remain speculative although they are apparently present in the blood (7).

A new hypothesis proposes that peptides, oligonucleotides, and other small metabolites produced by the cancer are responsible for the genesis of the anorexia (32). They produce the anorexia through a peripheral effect on neuroendocrine cells and neuroreceptors and through a direct effect on hypothalamic and other central nervous system sensor and responder cells.

The symptom of early satiety is an intriguing one although the mechanism remains unexplained. In the course of the disease, patients with cancer, despite being hungry at the beginning of the meal, start experiencing easy filling and an aversion to more food after the consumption of a small quantity of food.

The oligophagia that results from the anorexia and the early satiety plays a major role in the progressive weight loss and advancing cachexia of cancer, but as we shall see later, the decreased food intake alone cannot account entirely for the progressive tissue wasting.

INCREASED ENERGY EXPENDITURE

Mider and co-workers (33) demonstrated that rats in which Walker carcinoma 256 grew progressively lost more calories than their pair-fed noncancerous controls of the same age and initial weight. Kleiber and Chernikoff (34) showed that rats with a spontaneous breast tumor had an elevation of the metabolic rate per unit weight. Because the tumor had a relatively low metabolic rate, the increase in total rate did not result from the metabolism of the tumor itself. Following Walker tumor transplant, Pratt and Putney (35) observed an abrupt increase in total energy expenditure above control period levels in all animals that subsequently showed tumor growth. The increase in total energy expenditure became apparent almost immediately after tumor transplantation and before any tumor could be palpated. The authors state that the total energy expenditure is made up of three major components:

1. the resting basal energy cost, which is increased in the presence of growing tumor,
2. the energy cost of movement and activity, and
3. the energy cost of food utilization (35).

The spontaneous motor activity of the cancer-bearing animal actually declines during the tumor growth (36). Increased oxygen consumption of the tumor-bearing animals was also demonstrated with a more precise apparatus by Bramante and co-workers (37). Therefore, it appears that following the tumor transplantation, a process is initiated within the body that results in increased energy requirements (38).

In humans, one of the first reports was that of Wallersteiner, who studied energy metabolism in afebrile patients with advanced cancer (39). Approximately 50% of the patients had elevated metabolic rates while only two of the 33 patients studied had reduced metabolic rates. Although surgical removal of the carcinoma resulted in a reduction of the basal metabolic rate in one patient, recurrence of the tumor was always accompanied by an increased expenditure of energy. Comparable findings of frequently increased metabolic rates have been reported by others (38,40,41). Terepka's and Waterhouse's study (42), especially, provided more conclusive evidence that the caloric expenditure in some cancer patients is increased, and that the quantity of malignant tissue present does not appear to account for the increased values obtained.

In contrast to these data, there are very few reports in the literature of significantly low basal metabolic rates in patients with extensive cancer involvement.

In order to explain the increased energy expenditure, Fenninger and Mider considered two possibilities (43,44). First, the growth of malignant tissue proceeds continuously throughout the entire day in contrast to the diurnal periodicity of the metabolic activity of normal tissues and their periodic reduction of caloric expenditure, and consequently, the metabolism of the growing tumor imposes greater energy demands than the normal tissues. However, the contribution of the tumor to the total increment of energy expenditure is small because it has been shown that the metabolic rate of the tumor is relatively low as compared to the increased energy of the host (34).

Second, a selective removal of nutrients by the tumor results in alterations in the pathways of the intermediary metabolism of the host, forcing the host to use more expensive pathways in terms of energy. Mider further suggested that some biochemical reactions previously available to the host might be denied to him since the metabolites involved have already been utilized by the tumor (44). However, selective nutrient

utilization or destruction by the tumor leading to deficit of that particular nutrient for the host has not yet been documented. Furthermore, the
hyperalimentation experiments show that even though the metabolic
pool and the nutrient supply are augmented during forced feeding, the
abundance of nutrients frequently does not result in decreased energy
expenditure.

That the tumor induces an alteration in the oxidative and the energy
conserving systems of the host was another interesting hypothesis considered in the past (45). A substance was found in the 25,000 × g super-
natant of homogenate from the Novikoff hepatoma of the rat that could
uncouple the oxidative phosphorylation of normal liver mitochondria
(46). Such substances have also been demonstrated in the serum of
sarcoma-bearing rats in an in vitro study of oxidative phosphorylation of
normal liver mitochondria (47). When liver mitochondria from rats
bearing Walker carcinoma 256(48) and from mice bearing Krebs-2 carcinoma (45) were studied in vitro, no impairment in the oxidative phosphorylation was detected. However, others reported an uncoupling of
phosphorylation from oxidation in liver and kidney mitochondria of a
sarcoma-bearing rat in an in vitro assay (49). Nevertheless, there are no
in vivo studies available to show that increased energy expenditure of
the tumor-bearing animal is the result of some alteration in the energy-
yielding reactions and the coupling mechanisms of the host tissues.

Healthy subjects with decreased alimentation usually demonstrate decreased metabolic rates (50). Cancer patients, in contrast, may show
increased oxygen consumption despite their falling caloric intake.

Semistarvation causes a decrease in oxygen consumption, resulting in
diminished ATP requirements since the formation of glycogen, fatty
acids, and triglycerides that result from transient excesses of foodstuffs
is diminished (51). However, in patients with cancer in the postabsorp-
tive state, Waterhouse demonstrated that oxidative metabolism persisted
at increased rates (51). Thus, why the tumor-bearing host does not adapt
its energy metabolism to a state of semistarvation remains unexplained.

NITROGEN LOSS

Animal Studies

The nitrogen balance of rats bearing transplanted sarcoma was studied
in 1928 by Mischetschenko and Fomenko (52). They observed that the
rat carcasses actually lost weight as the neoplasm grew, and estimating
the nitrogen intake as sufficiently large to provide for weight increment

to the carcass, they thought that this indicated that the neoplastic tissues obtained foodstuffs from normal tissues.

Mider and co-workers demonstrated that the nitrogen content of a large Walker carcinoma 256 exceeded the amount of nitrogen stored by the host during the period of tumor growth and concluded that part of the nitrogen contained in a tumor must have been derived from the host's body. Their data indicated that cancerous rats break down normal protoplasm to provide building blocks for neoplastic tissue (43,53,54). Sherman and co-workers demonstrated that the tissues that lose nitrogen during caloric starvation are the ones that lose nitrogen during a tumor growth (55).

The concentration of amino nitrogen was found elevated in the blood of tumor-bearing mice (56–58) and decreased in the muscle (58). Sassenrath and Greenberg (59,60) observed not only some changes in concentration of free amino acids in host tissues but also an increased rate of metabolism of several of the amino acids in the tumor-bearing animal. Amino acids released by host tissues to the metabolic pool are used by the tumor for its growth. Bapson and Winnik (61) even presented evidence to support the view that protein is transferred from the body tissues of Walker carcinoma rats to the growing tumor without prior complete hydrolysis to free amino acids.

These animal studies demonstrated conclusively that when the dietary intake becomes inadequate, nitrogen is relinquished by the host tissues and is taken by the tumor. With isotopically labeled amino acids, it has been demonstrated that for the most part this is a one-way passage from the host to the tumor (54). However, the tumor can grow even when the diet contains no proteins (62).

Observations in Humans

Muller in 1889 compared the total nitrogen excretion of patients with advanced cancer to that of patients who, for various reasons, ate little or no food. The majority of the cancer patients excreted appreciably more nitrogen than the reference starved group (63). Co and associates observed that cancer patients on voluntary intake of hospital food were usually in negative nitrogen balance (64).

In general, patients with cancer may display nitrogen metabolism ranging all the way from positive to very negative nitrogen balance (65–67). But even when they are in positive nitrogen balance, the nitrogen may be retained by the tumor, while the host may be actually in negative balance.

In the blood of patients with leukemia and cancer, amino acid nitrogen (68–71), protein split products, "proteose" (72), and amino acids (73–75) have been found elevated. Abnormalities were observed also in the urine excretion of various amino acids in patients with malignant neoplastic diseases (76–77). It appears that the free amino acid pattern of the blood and tissues of the patient is altered during the growth of the tumor, most probably as a primary effect of cancer and not secondary to the decreased protein intake. In accordance with this is the finding that the total amino acid nitrogen in the blood of cancer patients is elevated, by contrast with the decreased level in individuals starved for prolonged periods (78).

Hyperalimentation of the cancer patient can temporarily correct the negative nitrogen balance (42,79,80). This can occur in spite of a negative caloric balance because again the nitrogen is stored mainly by the cancer. During forced feeding there was an initial retention of a significant quantity of nitrogen and phosphorus, but frequently the nitrogen balance gradually approached equilibrium and then moved toward a negative balance (42).

Hypoalbuminemia is a well-known and common clinical feature of cancer (81–83). With hyperalimentation, cancer patients may demonstrate weight gain but the plasma albumin may remain low (84). The pathogenesis of hypoalbuminemia appears to be a primary defect in albumin synthesis (85) and this probably represents the generalized disturbance of the protein synthesis in the patient with malignant disease (86).

Levenson and Watkin (87) pointed out that nitrogen turnover and loss seem to be proportional to the activity of the cancer and the practical answer to nitrogen loss is not protein feeding but reversal of the trend of the disease.

LOSS OF FAT

Experimental and Clinical Observations

Mider and co-workers demonstrated that with the progressive growth of the Walker carcinoma, rats lost significantly more total lipid than pair-fed controls of the same age, weight, and sex (88). Changes in lipid content of the tumor-bearing host have been seen with several types of experimental approaches (89–92). A decrease in the neutral fat content of the carcass, skeletal muscles, and intestine of the tumor-bearing animals and an increase in the phospholipids and free cholesterol content of carcass, skeletal muscle, and intestine have been observed. Because of mobilization of fat from the stores, blood taken during the active growth of the tumor was generally lipemic. The lipemia subsided terminally and it was then found that the fat stores were empty (91). Hence it was concluded that fat was mobilized to meet increased caloric requirements of the host.

Profound alterations of the lipid metabolism of tumor-bearing animals have been reported by several investigators in various tumor systems (93–96).

The clinical manifestation of a marked loss of adipose tissue that accompanies progressing cancer is the most striking picture of the patient with advanced cancer. The progressive emaciation, the phthisis, that was a characteristic of active tuberculosis in the past, today has become a hallmark of cancer.

Extensive work in humans by Watkin demonstrated a rapid reduction per unit time in the total quantity of body fat in the cancer patient (97). The caloric expenditure was elevated, the caloric deficit was not corrected by hyperalimentation, and the hypermetabolism was associated with an increased utilization of fat per unit time.

A comparison of adipose tissue of patients with breast cancer to controls, through the use of gas liquid phase chromatography, demonstrated no significant differences in the percent composition of the major fatty acid with a carbon chain length of C–12 to C–18 (98). However, a significant increase in plasma unesterified fatty acid concentrations was noted in a group of patients with neoplastic disease (99). The unesterified fatty acids originate primarily from adipose tissue and supply fats to tissues for oxidative metabolism (100,101). Fat is an excellent source of energy, and a good correlation has been demonstrated between energy expenditure and fat loss in tumor-bearing rats.

The lipid lost from the body during the tumor growth must be burned completely, for no significant ketosis has been demonstrated in tumor-bearing animals (33). Furthermore, in the cancer patient, the rate of removal of infused lipids from the blood appears to be increased (102). The intriguing question, then, is how can the tumor induce the host to mobilize fat for energy metabolism.

Fat mobilizing substances have been isolated from the urine of fasted animals and humans. Identified as peptides, these substances could first mobilize fat from the fat depots, second, increase the total metabolic turnover of fat in the animals, and third, increase the total amount of fat in the liver. Initially, it was thought that they also had anorexigenic properties, but since then peptides with anorexigenic and peptides with lipolytic properties have been separated and partially purified (103–112).

It is of interest that even during the early investigations, fat mobilizing activity was detected in the urine of patients with widespread malignant disease, even in those with a normal food intake (104).

At first, it was thought that such peptides were of pituitary origin, but subsequent work demonstrated that they were produced even in the absence of the pituitary gland (109–110). Peptides with lipid mobilizing activity have been detected not only in pituitary extracts (113–114), but also in hypothalamic extracts of mammalian species, including man (115–116). Furthermore, lipolytic activity has been reported in extracts from various other parts of the brain (117–118).

To explain the striking depletion of body lipid stores during the course of tumor growth, Leibelt and co-workers (119) and others suggested that the neoplastic cells may elaborate a lipid mobilizing substance.

ALTERED CARBOHYDRATE METABOLISM

The carbohydrate metabolism of the malignant neoplastic cell differs markedly from that of the normal cell (120–123), but for this chapter it is the altered carbohydrate metabolism of the tumor-free tissues of animals and patients with cancer that is of interest. This altered carbohydrate metabolism is connected to the derangement of protein and lipid metabolism in the tumor-bearing host. Actually, Gold proposed that a greatly augmented pathway of gluconeogenesis in the cancer host is the major cause of energy loss and cachexia (122).

Low liver glycogen levels in tumor-bearing animals has frequently been reported (124–126). No differences in phosphorylase activity could be detected between the livers of the tumor-bearing and control animals (127), although tumor-bearing mice and rats given a glucose load deposited less glycogen in the liver than control animals (128).

Glicksman and Rawson, using a standard oral glucose tolerance test, found that in 628 patients with cancer 36.7% had diabetic glucose tolerance curves versus only 9.3% of the controls (129). Marks and Bishop demonstrated that the intravenously administered glucose had a disappearance rate in cancer patients significantly lower than in the controls ($K = 2.20 \pm 0.90$ for the former, versus 4.16 ± 1.52 %/minute for the latter (130)). The fasting blood sugar in the cancer group did not differ significantly from that of the controls, and the same authors in another study demonstrated that patients with neoplastic disease had a decreased sensitivity to insulin (131). This decreased sensitivity and various other mechanisms have been proposed to explain the altered carbohydrate metabolism of the cancer patient (132).

Waterhouse and Kemperman reported that when glucose was administered, the normal metabolic adjustments were severely limited in patients with metastatic cancer (132). Carbon dioxide production from labeled glucose showed only a modest increase, labeled free fatty acid oxidation decreased less than normal, and CO_2 production from unlabeled substances was unchanged from that found in the fasting state.

In a recent study of patients with breast cancer, we demonstrated that the mean insulinogenic index, representing the quantity of insulin secreted per unit of glycemic stimulus, was lower than the reported normal controls (133). This index of insulinogenic reserve is a ratio of the enhancement of circulating insulin above fasting value over the increase of glycemic stimulus from the fasting value. Thus, in the patient with advanced cancer, it appears that the insulin response to glucose may be impaired.

WATER AND ELECTROLYTE ABNORMALITIES

Several investigators have detected the water and sodium abnormalities in the carcass of tumor-bearing animals and the topic has been reviewed by Costa (120). Subsequently, Morrison reported not only that the water content is increased but that salt supplements cause further water retention (134).

Body composition changes in patients with advanced cancer were evaluated by Waterhouse and Craig (135), who used a more direct calculation of changes in total body water employing the dilution of deuterium oxide (D_2O). They demonstrated that cancer patients lost body fat but gained in total body water, which was shared by the intracellular and extracellular compartments of the body. Furthermore, it was shown that even after hyperalimentation, the weight gained was predominantly due to an accumulation of large quantities of intracellular fluid (42). In this respect, patients with advanced cancer differ from individuals who have an insufficient caloric intake due to other causes, as in the latter situation, only extracellular fluid is increased.

The most common clinical electrolyte abnormality in advanced cancer patients is hyponatremia. This is rather difficult to correct and, once corrected, it is difficult to maintain a normal serum sodium level for long periods in the face of advancing cachexia.

BODY WEIGHT LOSS

To the patient and relatives, the most obvious feature of cancer cachexia is the weight loss. This manifestation is the end result of all the metabolic abnormalities previously described.

In just a short period after innoculation with a tumor, the total weight of the animal (animal plus tumor) starts increasing (136–137), and continues to increase up to a few days before death, when the total weight starts decreasing (138). The weight of the carcass (animal minus tumor) might remain stable or even increase for a very short initial period, but then progressively decreases (136–137). This initial increase in the carcass weight is the result of an increase in the water content of the body of tumor-bearing animals, because the animal carcass contains less nitrogen and less fat (139).

In the tumor-bearing animal, the alimentary canal weight maintains the normal ratio to total body weight (136). The heart shows hypertrophy in most animals, and the liver in all (136,140,141). The dry liver to total animal weight ratio is greater than the normal values even when the estimated loss in carcass weight is added to the total body weight (142). At present, it remains unexplained why the liver gains weight in cancer when all other tissues lose weight, in contrast to starvation, where the liver, also, loses weight.

Although the anorexia and oligophagia are major contributory factors to the progressive weight loss, forced feeding, paired feeding, and caloric restriction experiments in tumor-bearing animals have established that malnutrition alone cannot account entirely for the progressive cachexia (143–146). In humans, too, hyperalimentation only temporarily reverses the tissue wasting process (42).

It is of interest, also, to contrast the effects of tumor growth with those resulting from pregnancy. In both cases, there is a rapid growth made possible by supply of nutrients by the host. While the pregnant rat shows a gain in carcass protein and in carcass weight, the tumor-bearing rat carcass may lose weight and protein (147) even with forced feeding. An obvious conclusion is that the effect of pregnancy on the metabolism of the host is different from the effects of the tumor on the host.

ANEMIA

The etiology of anemia in the advanced cancer patient is multifactorial. A decrease in hemoglobin and red blood cell production, an increased red blood cell destruction, and an increased red blood cell loss may result for various reasons and contribute to the genesis of anemia. The anemia may result in tissue hypoxia, the role of which, if any, in cancer cachexia remains unknown. Actually, the pathogenesis of cardiac cachexia has been attributed entirely to cellular hypoxia (148).

ASTHENIA

Asthenia is characterized by marked weakness, general debility, decreased effort tolerance, and a gradual progressive fading of most of the functions of the host. The muscle wasting and the decreased muscle use contribute to the asthenia and a marked weakness of the respiratory muscle may result in weak bellows action of the thorax with a tendency to areas of atelectasis in both lungs, pneumonitis, and death.

OTHER HOST METABOLIC ABNORMALITIES

Several other changes take place in the host with an undetermined role at present in the genesis of cancer cachexia: deficiencies of several vitamins in host tissues have been reported (149); changes in the content and concentration of various minerals in the plasma and in the tissues of the host have been documented (120), and hormonal changes in the cancer patients have been described. Although the role of endocrine dysfunction in the genesis of cachexia has not been studied adequately, the presence of cachexia and malnutrition in the host induces significant alterations of the function of the endocrine system. For instance, it is known that the normal secretion of many polypeptide hormones is affected by the starvation and the plasma concentration of a number of specific nutrients (150).

The presence of cancer also alters significantly the activity of various host enzymes (128,151,152). Alterations of the activity of enzymes of protein, carbohydrate, lipid, and nucleic acid metabolism and of other enzymes are part of this profound derangement of the host metabolism. On the other hand, some enzymes of the host are not affected by the presence of cancer (128).

DISCUSSION OF PATHOGENESIS

For the sake of simplicity, energy expenditure, protein and lipid loss, and carbohydrate and other metabolic abnormalities have been discussed separately. Naturally, all these aspects of the host metabolism are interconnected, interdependent, and mutually influential.

The crucial question is how the tumor affects the host metabolism and induces the anorexia, the increased energy expenditure, the alterations in the metabolism of protein, lipid, carbohydrate, and other compounds that together lead to the cancer cachexia and death.

It is well established that frequently cancers produce peptides and other small molecules (153) as a result of derepression of various genomes (154). Novel and common peptides in the blood and urine of animals and patients with malignant neoplastic growth have been demonstrated repeatedly (155–158). Several of these peptides were not found in healthy controls or in patients with other diseases (155). Such peptides may appear early in the course of the disease or later as the cancer progresses and clonal evolution of tumor cell population takes place (159).

Novel and common peptides and other small molecules produced by the tumor may modify the activity of host enzymes through allosteric transitions, activations, and inactivations (160) of various enzymes in the tissues of the host (160). It is well known that the activity of enzymes may be modulated by many kinds of small molecules that have the ability to affect the catalytic activity of protein by binding to it at a molecular site some distance from the active site. This type of control mechanism does not even require change in the total amount of enzyme protein (160).

Through this allosteric effect, alterations in the metabolic pattern of the host and changes in various metabolic equilibria and concentrations of metabolites take place. The cancer, by producing these low molecular weight metabolites, throws the metabolism of the host into a chaotic state, activating or inactivating usual biochemical reactions without a purpose, need, or plan for the host. This increased metabolic activity results in an increased energy expenditure, an inability to lower basal metabolic rates despite the semistarvation, and the release of intermediate metabolites that enter the metabolic pool of the host and are trapped and used primarily by the tumor which is geared mainly to growth. The tumor, through convergence of enzyme activity, limits biochemical reactions to those essential for growth (161), and becomes less vulnerable for activation of unnecessary biochemical reactions by the small molecules it produces.

The small molecules produced by the cancer may also be responsible for the anorexia and the lipolysis, by directly or indirectly inducing the brain to produce anorexigenic and lipolytic peptides.

Work from several laboratories has suggested the possibility that low molecular weight peptides may have important direct effects on brain function (162). Adrenocorticotrophic hormone and melatonin can influence the behavior of laboratory animals (163,164). Injection of angiotensin II into the anterior diencephalon causes the rats to drink water

(165). Low molecular weight peptides have also been implicated in the regulation of sleep (166) and memory (167).

Martin and co-workers (162) advanced the hypothesis that hypothalamic peptidergic neurons may be involved in the formation of a diffuse neural network that terminates in widespread regions of the central nervous system. They postulated that these hypothalamic peptides may have a great importance in central nervous system biological regulation. One could hypothesize that peptides and other small molecules released from the cancer can have a direct effect on neurosecretory cells in the hypothalamus, pituitary, and other parts of the brain, stimulating the release of anorexigenic and lipolytic peptides. The anorexigenic peptides are responsible for the anorexia. The lipolytic peptides cause lipolysis and utilization of fatty acids for energy production for the increased caloric needs of the host resulting from its chaotic metabolism. Experimental proof for my hypothesis is not available at present.

There is, of course, a certain percentage of patients with cancer who never develop cachexia, and at death still have adequate stores of adipose tissue and adequate muscle mass. This can be seen even after a long presence of metastatic disease. An explanation for this phenomenon could be that this particular cancer did not produce peptides and other small molecules and did not affect significantly the metabolism of the host.

While the pathogenesis of cancer cachexia described above refers to the mechanism directly related to the growth of the tumor, there are additional major indirect contributory factors. Such factors result from the complications of the disease itself, and from the effects and complications of surgery, radiotherapy, chemotherapy, and immunotherapy. The major ones are: maldigestion, malabsorption, gastrointestinal protein loss, albuminuria, malignant effusions, hemorrhage, necrosis and ulcerations, infections, and impaired function of various organs. Furthermore, cancer patients may have other concomitant metabolic diseases such as diabetes mellitus, chronic renal disease, chronic liver disease, and alcoholism that may adversely affect the nutrition of the host.

Patients with advanced cancer, especially those receiving radiotherapy and chemotherapy, have impaired humoral and cellular immunologic responsiveness to challenge. The role of impaired immunologic mechanisms in the genesis of the cancer cachexia remains unknown. It is, however, well known that with immunopathologic conditions such as the runting syndrome, tissue wasting may be a prominent feature.

A detailed description of the etiology and the manifestations of the indirect factors and complications that contribute to the development of cachexia by affecting the nutrition and the metabolism of the host is beyond the scope of this chapter.

MANAGEMENT OF CANCER CACHEXIA

The only effective management of cancer cachexia is surgical, radiotherapeutic, and chemotherapeutic cure or prolonged control of the cancer. Prevention or control of complications of the cancer and of the treatment may also arrest or delay the development of the cachexia syndrome.

As a result of the pessimistic attitude prevailing in the nutritional management of the cancer patient in the past, an aggressive nutritional support was rarely attempted in the presence of cachexia. Lately, however, maintenance and improvement of the advanced cancer patient's nutritional state is being recognized more and more as a major aspect of the supportive management (168).

Early in the management of recurrent or metastatic cancer, a complete nutritional history should be obtained, while an assessment of the nutritional status by simple and practical methods and basic clinical skills (169) should be done periodically throughout the course of the disease.

The total caloric intake, the meal patterns, and food composition can be adversely affected not only by physical infirmities but by psychological and emotional disturbances as well. Thus, the nutritional management of the patient should include compassion, understanding, and emotional support in addition to the antidepressant drugs, tranquilizers, hypnotics, antiemetics, and analgesics, when needed.

Various aspects and approaches for the enteral and parenteral alimentation and hyperalimentation of the advanced cancer patient are presented by other authors in this volume.

Although at present there is no conclusive evidence that aggressive nutritional management significantly prolongs the survival of the cachectic cancer patient, it may improve the quality of life, and increase the tolerance to chemotherapy and other therapeutic modalities.

REFERENCES

1. J. D. Hardy, *Surg. Clin. North Am.,* **42**, 305 (1962).
2. G. E. Chisholm, *Ann. N.Y. Acad. Sci.,* **230**, 403 (1974).
3. J. R. Bignall, *Lancet,* **1**, 786 (1955).
4. S. Warren, *Am. J. Med. Sci.,* **184**, 610 (1932).

5. H. Nebenzahl, *Progr. Med.*, **46**, 1926 (1932).

6. H. Donovan, *Proc. R. Soc. Med.*, **47**, 27 (1953).

7. A. Theologides, *Ann. N.Y. Acad. Sci.*, **230**, 14 (1974).

8. B. K. Anand, *Physiol. Rev.*, **41**, 677 (1961).

9. M. I. Grossman, *Ann. N.Y. Acad. Sci.*, **63**, 76 (1955).

10. H. D. Janowitz, *Am. J. Med.*, **25**, 327 (1958).

11. M. I. Grossman, *Am. J. Clin. Nutr.*, **8**, 562 (1968).

12. B. C. Walkie, H. A. Jordan, and E. Stellar, *J. Comp. Physiol. Psychol,* **68**, 327 (1968).

13. S. Lepkovsky, R. Lyman, D. Fleming, M. Nagumo, and M. M. Dimick, *Am. J.Physiol.*, **188**, 327 (1957).

14. A. E. Harper and H. E. Spivey, *Am. J. Physiol.*, **193**, 483 (1958).

15. J. R. Brobeck, *Yale J. Biol. Med.*, **20**, 545 (1948).

16. J. L. Strominger and J. R. Brobeck, *Yale J. Biol. Med.*, **25**, 383 (1953).

17. J. Mayer, *N. Engl. J. Med.*, **249**, 13 (1953).

18. J. Mayer, *Ann. N.Y. Acad. Sci.*, **63**, 15 (1955).

19. J. Mayer, *Clin. Res. Proc.*, **5**, 123 (1957).

20. G. C. Kennedy, *Proc. R. Soc. Lond. (Biol)*, **140**, 578 (1953).

21. S. M. Mellinkoff, M. Frankland, D. Boyle, and M. Greipel, *J. Appl. Physiol.*, **8**, 535 (1956).

22. S. M. Mellinkoff, *Ann. Rev. Physiol.*, **19**, 175 (1957).

23. M. I. Grossman, G. M. Cummins, and A. C. Ivy, *Am. J. Physiol.*, **149**,100 (1947).

24. J. Mayer, *Am. J. Clin. Nutr.*, **8**, 547 (1960).

25. F. X. Hauserberger and B. C. Hauserberger, *Am. J. Clin. Nutr.*, **8**,671 (1960).

26. W. M. Hunter, J. A. R. Friend, and J. A. Strong, *J. Endocrinol.*, **34**,139 (!().

27. W. M. Hunter and W. M. Rigal, *J. Endocrinol.*, **34**, 147 (1966).

28. S. B. Penick and L. Hinkle, Jr., *Am. J. Clin. Nutr.*, **13**, 110 (1963).

29. A. V. Schally, T. W. Redding, H. W. Lucien, and J. Mayer, *Science,* **157**,210 (1967).

30. N. R. Defny, R. H. Jacob, and E. D. Jacobson, *Clin. Res.*, **36**, 45A (1975).

31. A. M. Ugolev and V. G. Kassil, *Usp. Sovrem. Biol.*, **51**, 352 (1961).

32. A. Theologides, *Am. J. Clin. Nutr.*, **29**, 552 (1976).

33. G. B. Mider, L. D. Fenninger, F. L. Haven, and J. J. Morton, *Cancer Res.*, **11**, 731 (1951).

34. M. Kleiber and T. Chernikoff, *J. Gerontol.*, **11**, 140 (1956).

35. J. W. Pratt and F. K. Putney, *J. Natl. Cancer Inst.*, **20**, 173 (1958).

36. S. D. Morrison, *J. Natl. Cancer Inst.*, **51**, 1535 (1973).

37. P. O. Bramante, A. S. Nunn, M. C. Steiner, and D. E. Beaulieu, *J. Appl. Physiol.*, **18**, 216 (1963).

38. G. B. Mider, *Cancer Res.*, **11**, 821 (1951).

39. E. Wallersteiner, *Deutsch. Arch. Klin. Med.*, **116**, 145 (1914).

40. J. B. Murphy, J. H. Means, and J. C. Aub, *Arch. Intern. Med.*, **19**,890 (1917).

41. S. Silver, P. Poroto, and E. B. Crohn, *Arch. Intern. Med.*, **85**,479 (1950).

42. A. R. Terepka and C. Waterhouse, *Am. J. Med.*, **20**, 225 (1956).

43. L. D. Fenninger and G. B. Mider, *Adv. Cancer Res.*, **2**, 229 (1954).

44. G. B. Mider, *Can. Cancer Conf.*, **1**, 120 (1955).

45. T. M. Devlin and G. Costa, *Proc. Soc. Exp. Biol. Med.*, **116**, 1095 (1964).

46. T. M. Devlin and M. P. Pruss, *Fed. Proc.*, **17**, 211 (1958).

47. G. Nanni and A. Casu, *Experientia*, **17**, 402 (1961).

48. A. A. Greene, *Cancer Res.*, **20**, 233 (1960).

49. G. Nanni, *Sperimentale*, **111**, 55 (1961).

50. A. Keyes, J. Brozek, A. Henschel, D. Mickelson, and H. L. Taylor, *The Biology of Human Starvation,* University of Minnesota Press, Minneapolis (1950).

51. C. Waterhouse, *Ann. N.Y. Acad. Sci.*, **230**, 86 (1974).

52. I. P. Mischetschenko and M. M. Fomenko, *Z. Krebsforsch*, **27**, 427 (1928).

53. G. B. Mider, H. Tesluk, and J. J. Morton, *Acta Un. Int. Cancr.*, **6**, 409 (1948).

54. G. B. Mider, *Ann. Rev. Med.*, **4**, 187 (1953).

55. C. D. Sherman, Jr., J. J. Morton, and G. B. Mider, *Cancer Res.*, **10**, 374 (1950).

56. M. M. ElMehary, *Brit. J. Cancer*, **4**, 95 (1950).

57. V. H. Auerbach and H. A. Waisman, *Cancer Res.*, **18**, 536 (1958).

58. C. Wu and J. M. Bauer, *Cancer Res.*, **20**, 848 (1960).

59. E. N. Sassenrath and D. M. Greenberg, *Cancer Res.*, **14**, 563 (1954).

60. D. M. Greenberg and E. N. Sassenrath, *Cancer Res.*, **15**, 620 (1955).

61. A. L. Bapson and T. Winnik, *Cancer Res.*, **14**, 606 (1954).

62. F. R. White and M. Belkin, *J. Natl. Cancer Inst.*, **5**, 261 (1945).

63. F. Muller, *Ztschr. Klin. Med.*, **16**, 496 (1889).

64. T. Co, N. H. Kuo, M. Chuachiaco, R. Rosh, and J. H. Mulholland, *Surg. Clin. North Am.*, **29**, 449 (1949).

65. C. Waterhouse, L. D. Fenninger, and E. H. Keutmann, *Cancer*, **4**, 500 (1951).

66. L. D. Fenninger, C. Waterhouse, and E. H. Keutmann, *Cancer*, **6**, 930 (1953).

67. D. M. Watkin, *Am. J. Clin. Nutr.*, **9**, 446 (1961).

68. A. Goldfeder, *Z. Krebsforsch*, **40**, 394 (1934).

69. S. L. Malowan, *Archiv. Tierheilkunde*, **65**, 279 (1932).

70. S. Okada and T. Hayashi, *J. Biol. Chem.*, **51**, 121 (1922).

71. K. Sandiford, W. M. Boothly, and H. L. Giffin, *J. Biol. Chem.*, **55**, 23 (1923).

72. R. J. Winzler, D. Burk, and M. Hasselback, *J. Natl. Cancer Inst.*, **4**, 417 (1944).

73. J. J. Kelley and H. A. Weisman, *Blood*, **12**, 635 (1957).

74. S. LoBianco and I. Sala, *Lattanta*, **25**, 649 (1954).

75. H. A. Waisman, R. A. Pastel, and H. G. Poncher, *Pediatrics*, **10**, 653 (1952).

76. C. H. Eades, Jr. and R. L. Pollack, *J. Natl. Cancer Inst.*, **15**, 421 (1954).

77. C. Wiseman, R. F. McGregor, and K. B. McCredie, *Cancer*, **38**, 219 (1976).

78. O. E. Owen, P. Felig, A. P. Morgan, J. Wahren, and G. F. Cahill, Jr., *J. Clin. Invest.*, **48**, 574 (1969).

79. N. Bolker, *Am. J. Roentgenol.*, **69**, 839 (1953).

80. M. D. Pareira, E. J. Conrad, W. Hicks, and R. Elman, *Cancer*, **8**, 803 (1955).

81. F. Homburger and N. F. Young, *Blood*, **3**, 1460 (1948).

82. I. M. Ariel, *Surg. Gynecol. Obst.*, **88**, 185 (1949).

83. G. B. Mider, E. I. Alling, and J. J. Morton, *Cancer*, **3**, 56 (1950).

84. J. C. Peden, Jr., L. F. Bond, and M. Maxwell, *Am. J. Clin. Nutr.,* **5**, 305 (1957).

85. J. L. Steinfeld, *Cancer,* **13**, 974 (1960).

86. C. Waterhouse and A. R. Terepka, *Metabolism,* **8**, 160 (1959).

87. S. M. Levenson and D. M. Watkin, *Fed. Proc.,* **181**, 1155 (1959).

88. G. B. Mider, C. D. Sherman, Jr., and J. J. Morton, *Cancer Res.,* **9**,222 (1949).

89. E. M. Boyd, M. L. Connell, and H. D. McEwen, *Can. J. Biochem.,* **30**,471 (1952).

90. H. D. McEwen, *Can. Cancer Conf.,* **1**, 149 (1955).

91. W. R. Bloor and F. L. Haven, *Cancer Res.,* **15**, 173 (1955).

92. E. M. Boyd, S. Jarzylo, and M. N. Shanas, *Cancer,* **13**, 850 (1960).

93. E. Schwenk and D. F. Stevens, *Cancer Res.,* **18**, 193 (1958).

94. J. A. Trew and R. W. Begg, *Cancer Res.,* **19**, 1014 (1959).

95. G. Costa and J. F. Holland, *Cancer Res.,* **22**, 1081 (1962).

96. G. Costa, K. Lyles, and L. Ullrich, *Cancer,* **38**, 1259 (1976).

97. D. M. Watkin, *Acta Un. Int. Cancr.,* **15**, 907 (1959).

98. W. T. Dabney, *J. Natl. Cancer Inst.,* **27**, 25 (1961).

99. T. S. Muller and D. M. Watkin, *J. Lab. Clin. Med.,* **57**, 95 (1961).

100. R. S. Gordon, Jr. and A. Cherkes, *J. Clin. Invest.,* **35**, 206 (1956).

101. R. S. Gordon, Jr., A. Cherkes, and H. Gates, *J. Clin. Invest.,* **36**,810, 1957.

102. C. Waterhouse and W. H. R. Nye, *Metabolism,* **10**, 403 (1961).

103. R. Weil and D. Stetten, Jr., *J. Biol. Chem.,* **168**, 129 (1947).

104. T. M. Chalmers, A. Keckwick, and G. L. S. Pawan, *Lancet,* **1**, 886(1958).

105. T. M. Chalmers, G. L. S. Pawan, and A. Kekwick, *Lancet,* **1**, 6 (1960).

106. T. Braun, P. Fabry, R. Petrasek, and J. Rudinger, *Experientia,* **19**,319 (1963).

107. J. A. F. Stevenson, D. M. Box, and A. J. Szlavko, *Proc. Soc. Exp. Biol. Med.,* **115**, 424 (1964).

108. J. R. Beaton, A. J. Szlavko, and J. A. F. Stevenson, *Can. J. Physiol. Pharmacol.,* **42**, 647 (1964).

109. J. A. F. Stevenson and J. R. Beaton, *Ann. N.Y. Acad. Sci.,* **131**,189 (1965).

110. J. R. Beaton and P. S. Uehara, *Can. J. Physiol. Pharmacol.,* **47**,291 (1969).

111. P. S. Uehara and J. R. Beaton, *Can. J. Physiol. Pharmacol.,* **48**,185 (1970).

112. M. Chretien and C. H. Li, *Can. J. Biochem.,* **45**, 1163 (1967).

113. D. Rudman, A. E. DelRio, L. A. Garcia, J. Barnett, C. H. Howard, W. Walker, and G. Moore, *Biochemistry,* **9**, 99 (1970).

114. Y. W. Lee and I. J. Lichton, *J. Nutr.,* **103**, 1616 (1973).

115. T. W. Redding and A. V. Schally, *Metabolism,* **19**, 641 (1970).

116. T. W. Redding, A. V. Schally, and A. Dupont, *Proc. 57th Ann. Meeting Endocrine Soc.,* abstr. 92 (1975).

117. L. Kadas and D. Dagy, *Endokrinologie,* **48**, 19 (1965).

118. C. R. Hollett, *Biochem. Biophys. Res. Commun.,* **32**, 48 (1968).

119. R. A. Liebelt, A. G. Liebelt, and H. M. Johnston, *Proc. Soc. Exp. Biol. Med.,* **138**, 482 (1971).

120. G. Costa, *Prog. Exp. Tumor Res.,* **3**, 321 (1963).

121. A. C. Aisenberg, *The Glycolysis and Respiration of Tumors,* Academic Press, New York (1961).

122. J. Gold, *Ann. N.Y. Acad. Sci.*, **230**, 103 (1974).

123. V. S. Shapot, *Adv. Cancer Res.*, **15**, 253 (1972).

124. A. Goldfeder, *Z. Krebsforsch*, **27**, 503 (1928).

125. N. F. Young, C. J. Kensler, L. Seki, and F. Homburger, *Proc. Soc. Exp. Biol. Med.*, **66**, 322 (1947).

126. E. S. Goranson, *Can. Cancer Conf.*, **1**, 330 (1955).

127. E. S. Goranson, J. McBride, and G. Weber, *Cancer Res.*, **14**, 227 (1954).

128. R. W. Begg, *Adv. Cancer Res.*, **5**, 1 (1958).

129. A. S. Glicksman and R. W. Rawson, *Cancer*, **9**, 1127 (1956).

130. P. A. Marks and J. Bishop, *Proc. Am. Assn. Cancer Res.*, **2**, 131 (1956).

131. P. A. Marks and J. Bishop, *Proc. Am. Assn. Cancer Res.*, **2**, 227 (1957).

132. C. Waterhouse and J. H. Kemperman, *Cancer Res.*, **31**, 273 (1971).

133. A. Theologides, R. B. McHugh, A. W. Lindall, and S. M. Hall, *Medical Pediatric Oncology*, in Press.

134. S. D. Morrison, *J. Natl. Cancer Inst.*, **52**, 869 (1974).

135. A. B. Craig, Jr. and C. Waterhouse, *Cancer*, **10**, 1106 (1957).

136. S. Medigrezeanu, *Proc. R. Soc. Lond. (Biol)*, **82**, 286 (1910).

137. J. A. Murray, *Imperial Cancer Research Fund, London*, 68 (1908).

138. C. S. McEwen and D. L. Thomson, *Brit. J. Exp. Pathol.*, **14**, 384 (1933).

139. M. S. Rechogl, Jr., F. Grantham, and R. E. Greenfield, *Cancer Res.*, **21**,238 (1961).

140. A. L. Babson, *Cancer Res.*, **14**, 89 (1954).

141. E. H. Yeakel, *Cancer Res.*, **8**, 392 (1948).

142. A. Theologides and C. H. Pegelow, *Proc. Soc. Exp. Biol. Med.*, **134**,1104 (1970).

143. A. G. Stewart and R. W. Begg, *Cancer Res.*, **13**, 556 (1953).

144. R. W. Begg, and T. E. Dickinson, *Cancer Res.*, **11**, 409 (1951).

145. R. W. Begg, *Can. Cancer Conf.*, **1**, 237 (1955).

146. T. Sugimura, S. M. Birnbaum, M. Winitz, and J. P. Greenstein, *Arch. Biochem. Biophys.*, **81**, 439 (1959).

147. E. W. McHenry, *Can. Cancer Conf.*, **1**, 149 (1955).

148. J. G. Pittman and P. Cohen, *N. Engl. J. Med.*, **271**, 403 and 453 (1960).

149. A. Theologides, *Minn. Med.*, **58**, 875 (1975).

150. R. A. Kreisberg, W. C. Owen, and A. M. Siegel, *Med. Clin. North Am.*, **54**, 1473 (1970).

151. J. P. Greenstein, *Biochemistry of Cancer*, 2nd ed., Academic Press, New York (1954), pp. 507–581.

152. A. Herzfeld and O. Greengard, *Cancer Res.*, **32**, 1826 (1972).

153. T. C. Hall, *Cancer Res.*, **34**, 2088 (1974).

154. E. H. Stonehill and A. Bendich, *Nature*, **228**, 370 (1970).

155. F. Hammarsten and B. M. Sandell, *Scand. J. Clin. Lab. Invest.*, **10**,42 (1958).

156. D. Rudman, A. DelRio, S. Akgun, and E. Frumin, *Am. J. Med.*, **46**,174 (1969).

157. L. H. Maurer and J. Pomeroy, *Clin. Res.*, **20**, 569 (1972).

158. R. Farbiszewski and W. Rzeczycki, *Experientia*, **30**, 855 (1974).

159. P. C. Nowell, *Science*, **194**, 23 (1976).

160. J. Monod, J. P. Changeux, and F. Jacob. *J. Mol. Biol.* **6**, 306 (1963).

161. J. P. Greenstein, *Cancer Res.*, **15**, 641 (1956).

162. J. B. Martin, L. P. Renaud, and P. Brazeau, *Lancet*, **2**, 393 (1975).

163. H. M. Greven and D. DeWied, *Progr. Brain Res.*, **39**, 429 (1973).

164. F. Anton-Tay, *Adv. Biochem. Psychopharmacol.*, **11**, 315 (1974).

165. J. T. Fitzsimons, *J. Physiol.*, **214**, 295 (1971).

166. J. R. Pappenheimer, V. Fench, and G. Koski *Proceedings of the 26th International Congress of Physiological Science,* 206 (1974).

167. G. Ungar, *Biochem. Pharmacol.*, **23**, 1553 (1974).

168. A. Theologides, Manuscript submitted for publication.

169. C. E. Butterworth and G. L. Blackburn, *Nutrition Today,* March/April, 8 (1975).

7

Specific Vitamin Deficiencies and Their Significance in Patients with Cancer and Receiving Chemotherapy

J. W. T. DICKERSON AND T. K. BASU

Division of Nutrition, Department of Biochemistry, University of Surrey, Guildford, Surrey, England

There is now a considerable amount of literature on the interactions of nutrition and cancer (1). Certain elements of our diet are thought to be involved in the etiology of cancer, and we have some understanding of the metabolic changes produced by the presence in the body of certain kinds of tumors. However, our knowledge about the relationships of specific nutrients, such as individual vitamins, to cancer in different sites is only beginning to emerge. Until recently, knowledge in this area had been derived from studies in experimental animals with nutrient requirements different from our own. Moreover, the animals usually carried transplantable tumors, or tumors evoked by the use of carcinogens, which may have little relation to tumors occurring in man.

It was for these reasons that we started to investigate the vitamin status and associated metabolism of patients with cancer in different sites. Our work has so far largely been restricted to vitamin A, thiamin, and ascorbic acid. This chapter deals mainly with our own work on patients; the literature on these three vitamins has been reviewed elsewhere (2).

VITAMIN A

A deficiency of vitamin A is thought to be associated with cancer of the stomach (3), the nasopharynx (4), and the lung (5). We have made a biochemical assessment of vitamin A status in patients with cancer in different sites including the breast, brain, respiratory organs, and alimentary tract. Our initial studies were made in patients with advanced disease who had all received surgery, radiotherapy, or a combination of these treatments (6). The patients ranged in age from 51 to 85 years. Those with tumors in the alimentary and respiratory tracts included both men and postmenopausal women, whereas all the patients with breast cancer were postmenopausal women, and all those with lung cancer were men. The controls used in this study were hospital patients of similar ages who did not have cancer, but had a variety of debilitating diseases such as tuberculosis, chronic bronchitis, coronary thrombosis, and hypertension. Estimates of body fat (7) were made in the cancer patients with the aid of skinfold calipers.

Patients with breast and brain tumors had a significantly higher percentage of body fat than patients of the same sex with tumors in other sites (Table 1). Patients with brain tumors had higher concentrations of vitamin A and β-carotene in their plasma than either the controls or the patients with cancer at other sites. Patients with cancer of the alimentary tract had lower concentrations of these two constituents than any of the other patients. The plasma cholesterol concentration paralleled the concentrations of vitamin A and β-carotene in the patients with tumors in the brain and alimentary tract, and in women with breast cancer the cholesterol level was higher than in women with cancer at other sites.

In all patients the concentrations of vitamin A were positively correlated with the concentrations of cholesterol. The low vitamin A and

Table 1   Body Fat and Plasma Vitamin A, β-carotene, and Cholesterol Concentrations in Patients with Advanced Cancer

	Fat (% body wt.)	Vitamin A	β-carotene	Cholesterol (mg/100 ml plasma)
		(μg/100 ml plasma)		
Alimentary tract (11)	12.5	30^c	49^c	158^c
Respiratory tract (6)	12.8	54	86	211
Breast (11)	30.0^b	60	82	231^b
Brain (7)	17.2^a	88^c	136^c	328^c
Controls (10)	—	59	92	197

[a] Significance of differences when compared with values for other sites shown, $p < 0.02$.
[b] Significance of differences when compared with values for other sites shown, $p < 0.01$.
[c] Significance of differences from control values shown, $p < 0.001$.

β-carotene values in patients with cancer of the alimentary tract may well be due to low fat diets which decrease the absorption of fat-soluble vitamins. The absorption of vitamin A from the gut is known to depend upon the presence of bile. It is therefore possible that the increased vitamin A levels in patients with brain tumors are due to increased absorption of the vitamin in the presence of excess intestinal bile acid derived from cholesterol. Brain tumors cause headache, and it seems possible that this may be exacerbated by the high plasma vitamin A levels. The cause of the hypercholesterolemia in the patients with brain tumors is not at present clear. It could be that they are the result of treatment, or that they are found only in patients with advanced disease. Further work is in hand to elucidate this matter.

Several studies have indicated that administration of vitamin A inhibits the development of squamous metaplasia and squamous cell tumors of the respiratory tract in experimental animals receiving carcinogens (8,9).

In a preliminary study (10), 28 patients, all cigarette smokers, diagnosed by chest X-ray, bronchoscopy, bronchial biopsy, and sputum cytology as having bronchial carcinoma, had lower plasma concentrations ($p < 0.01$) of vitamin A (45.6 μg/100 ml) than those with nonmalignant lung diseases (64.3 μg/100 ml) or healthy subjects (68.4 μg/100 ml). When the findings were grouped according to the histologic type of carcinoma, it was found that low values were present in those patients with squamous and oat cell carcinoma (39.6 and 36.3 μg/100 ml respectively) but not in those with large cell undifferentiated carcinoma (65.1 μg/100 ml). These findings do not, of course, establish a causal relationship. They are, however, in agreement with the findings in an epidemiological study by Bjelke (5) in Norway that showed a negative association between dietary vitamin A and lung cancer. This association recalls the report that in Holland a high incidence of bronchial carcinoma was found in individuals born in the winter months (11). Dijkstra sought to explain this association on the basis of the fact that at birth the plasma vitamin A level is low. If the baby is then fed on cow's milk which at that time of the year also has a low level, then the plasma level remains low at a critical time when the lungs are developing. As a result of this vitamin A deficiency, the bronchial mucosa may undergo metaplasia, later predisposing to squamous carcinoma when exposed to tobacco smoke (12). A possible biochemical explanation for a connection between vitamin A deficiency and lung carcinoma is provided by the work of Genta and co-workers (13), who showed that vitamin A deficiency enhanced the binding of metabolites of benzo(a)pyrene to tracheal epithelial DNA.

THIAMIN

In patients with advanced cancer we showed (14) that ten of a group of 38 patients studied had evidence of thiamin deficiency as shown by an elevated TPP value. The highest values for the TPP effect were found in those patients being treated with the cytotoxic drug 5-fluorouracil. In vitro studies with this drug suggested that it functions as a cocarboxylase antagonist. There was no question of a dietary deficiency of thiamin in these patients because all of them were receiving a supplementary multivitamin preparation. It is possible, however, that the vitamin was not absorbed from the intestine, since 5-fluorouracil has been reported to cause damage to the small intestine and malabsorption (15). However if this was the cause it might be expected that other cytotoxic drugs, such as methotrexate, which also caused changes in the intestinal mucosa, would be associated with low thiamin status. Methotrexate certainly does not appear to have the same effect (T. K. Basu, unpublished). It would therefore appear that 5-fluorouracil induces an increased requirement for thiamin.

The patients being treated with 5-fluorouracil in this study had advanced breast cancer. In a subsequent study (16) patients with early breast cancer were found to have significantly higher TPP values (14.5%) than those found in healthy age-matched controls (4.5%, $p <$ 0.01). These findings, together with those obtained in the previous study, suggest that the thiamin requirement may increase with progress of the tumor growth. However, it would be necessary to carry out a longitudinal study in order to prove this.

Patients with early bronchial carcinoma were also found to have TPP values (10.2%) that again were significantly higher than those of the healthy controls ($p <$ 0.01). These findings could be explained on the basis of a low dietary intake of thiamin. If this had been the explanation, however, we would not have expected to find a significantly elevated excretion of thiamin in the urine. Moreover, it seemed unlikely that increased excretion was responsible for the high TPP values since there was no significant relationship between these and the urinary excretion in the individual patients. We suggest therefore that the most likely explanation of the high TPP values, and of the apparent thiamin subnutrition in these patients is that conversion of thiamin to thiamin pyrophosphate was in some way impaired. Our previous work would suggest that this impairment is likely to be exacerbated by the administration of 5-fluorouracil. Unless it can be shown that a reduction in the phosphorylation of thiamin has an inhibitory action on tumor growth, our findings would indicate that patients with cancer may well benefit from administration of substantial thiamin supplements.

ASCORBIC ACID

Ascorbic acid plays a number of important roles in the body, and there is both direct and indirect evidence to suggest that it may be important in stress (17). There is also evidence that tissue stores of ascorbic acid are depleted in patients with malignant disease (18). We have been interested particularly in breast cancer. This is a common cause of death in women in Western countries. Furthermore, breast cancer almost invariably metastasizes to bone, and ascorbic acid plays a role in the hydroxylation of proline to form the hydroxyproline present in the collagen molecule, the principal constituent of the bone matrix.

We had access to 22 patients with advanced breast cancer and radiologically demonstrable skeletal metastases, and a group of 26 patients with malignant disease in other sites, such as brain, lung, throat, stomach, rectum, and cervix, but without skeletal involvement (19). As far as we could determine, all the patients had been receiving a similar diet, and additionally, the patients with breast tumors had been receiving vitamin supplements. Blood samples and fresh overnight urine samples were obtained from these patients, and from 10 healthy controls and 10 hospital patients in the same age range as the cancer patients, but with debilitating diseases such as tuberculosis, chronic bronchitis, and coronary thrombosis. Table 2 shows that the highest levels of leucocyte ascorbic acid were found in healthy subjects, and the lowest levels were found in the patients with breast cancer and skeletal metastases. The patients with nonmalignant disease and malignant disease without skeletal involvement had values that were intermediate.

The values for total urinary hydroxyproline followed an opposite

Table 2   Leucocyte Ascorbic Acid (LAA) Concentrations (μg/10^{8}WBC) and Total Urinary Hydroxyproline (Total UHP) Excretion (mg/g Creatinine) in Cancer Patients with and without Skeletal Metastases [a]

Cases (No.)	Sex	Age (years)	Osseous Deposits	LAA (μg/10^8 WBC)	Total UHP (mg/g creatinine)
Normal (10)	7M + 3F	58	—ve	33	16
Nonmalignant (10)	6M + 4F	64	—ve	21	46
Malignant nonbreast (26)	15M + 11F	62	—ve	19	46
Breast cancer	22F	66	+ve	12	135

[a]Values are means for the number of subjects shown.

pattern from those for leucocyte ascorbic acid, and were lowest in the healthy subjects and highest in the patients with breast cancer and skeletal metastases. Five patients with breast cancer and five patients with cancer in other sites were then given one gram of ascorbic acid by mouth, and urine collections were made at intervals of four hours over the next 12 hours. Table 3 shows that in the patients with breast cancer there was a fall in the excretion of hydroxyproline during the first four hours after the administration of ascorbic acid, and a lower level of excretion was maintained throughout the 12 hours of observation. These findings are in contrast to those in the other five patients whose leucocyte ascorbic acid levels had been normal, for oral ascorbic acid had no effect on the already low level of urinary hydroxyproline.

There can be no doubt that the increased excretion of hydroxyproline in patients with skeletal metastases is due to bone resorption and consequent extensive loss of bone matrix. Urinary hydroxyproline does, in fact, rise long before there are osseous deposits that can be detected radiologically (20). It may therefore be argued that it results from an increased rate of collagen degradation rather than from the activity of the tumor in the breast.

In these patients, the leucocyte ascorbic acid levels were low whereas the urinary hydroxyproline levels were high. This is a different situation from that reported in elderly people without clinical bone disease, where both levels are low (21). It is also different from the findings reported in

Table 3   Excretion of Hydroxyproline (UHP) by Patients with Advanced Breast Cancer and with Cancer at Other Sites after Administration of One Gram of Ascorbic Acid (AA)

Case No.	Site of tumor	Leucocyte ascorbic acid ($\mu g/10^8$ WBC)	UHP (mg/g creatinine) Hours after AA			
			0	4	8	12
1	Breast	9.8	84	50	46	52
2	Breast	6.0	160	72	54	49
3	Breast	5.8	260	65	13	22
4	Breast	7.2	112	78	56	42
5	Breast	10.3	91	47	43	33
6	Larynx	30.2	35	32	32	36
7	Pancreas	22.0	50	46	64	57
8	Bronchus	27.3	38	35	30	30
9	Rectum	20.2	40	32	30	30
10	Rectum	23.2	20	12	12	18

scorbutic guinea pigs, in which again low excretion of hydroxyproline accompanies low blood levels (22). There is evidence (23) that ascorbic acid may not only play a role in the synthesis of collagen but also protect the molecule from degradation. Our preliminary results suggest that comparatively large amounts of ascorbic acid may well do this in patients with skeletal metastases. An additional therapeutic, and possibly not unconnected, use of ascorbic acid in these patients is in the relief of bone pain (24). However, another possible explanation of the reported pain relief obtained with high doses of ascorbic acid is that it has an effect on tyrosine metabolism. It has been suggested that the high prolactin levels found in patients with breast cancer play a major role in its hormonal control. Prolactin levels are reduced by L-dopa (25,26), which reduces bone pain, and ascorbic acid is necessary for the in vivo synthesis of L-dopa from tyrosine.

The finding of a low level of ascorbic acid in the leucocytes of patients with breast cancer may form a link with two other facets of disturbed metabolism in these patients. We have already seen that plasma cholesterol levels were elevated. Cholesterol is converted to other steroids in the adrenal gland. This gland normally contains high concentrations of ascorbic acid, which plays a role in steroid synthesis. Various studies have indicated a possible relationship between abnormal levels of androgen and corticosteroid metabolites in the urine and plasma and the occurrence of breast cancer. In postmenopausal women with early breast cancer the finding (27) of low plasma levels of 11 hydroxycorticosteroids (Table 4) together with the elevated cholesterol levels would indicate a decreased synthesis of 11 OHCS by the adrenal gland which might well result from ascorbic acid depletion of the adrenal. Transformation to progesterone does not require ascorbic acid and in these patients the plasma level of progesterone was elevated. In premenopausal women, plasma progesterone may arise by secretion from the adrenal gland and ovary and also by extraglandular conversion from pregnenalone. It is not certain whether progesterone arises from these three sources in postmenopausal women. If it came from the adrenal this would represent a further aberration of adrenal metabolism which could in fact be responsible for the decreased plasma levels of 11OHCS.

Disturbances of tryptophan metabolism have been reported to be associated with alterations in urinary steroid excretion in patients with breast cancer (28), and in patients with advanced disease at various sites including breast, the excretion of 5 hydroxyindole acetic acid was increased while that of N-methylnicotinamide was reduced (29).

On the basis of these findings it seems possible to suggest that ascorbic

Table 4   Fecal Neutral Sterols and Bile Acids Excretion and Fecal 7α-dehydroxylase and Cholesterol Dehydrogenase Activity in Patients with Colon Cancer and Controls[a]

	Controls (31)	Colon Cancer Patients (31)
Neutral sterols (mg/g dry feces)		
Cholesterol	2.97	10.68
Coprostanol	12.44	17.53
Coprostanone	2.10	3.61
Cholestan-3β,5α,6β-triol	0.04	0.14
Total	17.55	31.96
Bile acids (mg/g dry feces)		
Cholic acid	0.32	0.54
Chenodeoxycholic acid	0.26	0.57
Deoxycholic acid	3.76	6.96
Lithocholic acid	3.13	6.41
Other bile acids[b]	3.38	5.19
Total	10.85	19.87
7α-dehydroxylase activity/100 mg dry feces	38.3	68.0
Cholesterol dehydrogenase activity/100 mg dry feces	20.8	55.5

[a]Data from Reddy and Wynder (48) and Mastromarino, Reddy, and Wynder (49).

[b]Other bile acids include ursodeoxycholic acid, 3-keto-5β-cholanic acid, 7-keto-lithocholic acid, 12-ketolithocholic acid, 7,12-diketolithocholic acid, and other microbially modified bile acids.

acid could play a key role in the metabolic changes found in patients with breast cancer (Fig. 1).

CONCLUSIONS

It is a matter of common observation and experience that the nutrition of the patient with cancer may be poor. Commonly, this is due to anorexia and low food intake. However, tumors of different kinds and

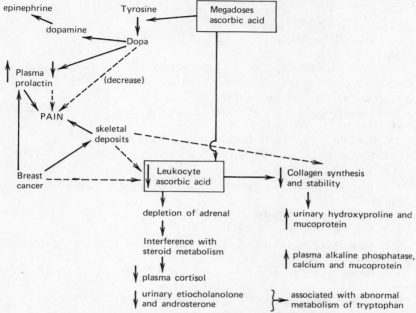

Suggested involvent of ascorbic acid in patients with advanced breast cancer

Figure 1. Suggested involvement of ascorbic acid in patients with advanced breast cancer.

at different sites may directly, or through associated hormone disturbances, increase the requirements for specific vitamins. Furthermore, an increased requirement for a specific vitamin may be induced by a cytotoxic drug, and amounts of certain vitamins greatly in excess of the normal requirement may well be useful in the management of patients with certain kinds of tumors.

ACKNOWLEDGMENTS

It is a pleasure to acknowledge the considerable help and encouragement that the authors have received from Mr. Ronald W. Raven, T.D., O.B.E., F.R.C.S., during the course of this work. Much of it was done while one of us (T.K.B.) was working in the Research Department of the Marie Curie Memorial Foundation.

REFERENCES

1. T. K. Basu, J. W. T. Dickerson, and D. C. Williams, *Ecology Food Nutr.*, **2**, 193, (1973).

2. T. K. Basu, *Oncology*. In press.

3. J. C. Abele, A. T. Gorham, G. T. Pack, and C. P. Rhoads, *J. Clin. Invest.*, **20**, 749 (1941).

4. E. L. Wynder and D. Hoffmann, "Nutrition and Cancer", *in* R. W. Raven and F. J. C. Roe, Eds., *The Prevention of Cancer*, Butterworths, London (1966), p. 11.

5. E. Bjelke, *Intl. J. Cancer*, **15**, 561 (1975).

6. T. K. Basu, R. W. Raven, J. W. T. Dickerson, and D. C. Williams, *Intl. J. Vit. Nutr. Res.*, **44**, 14 (1974).

7. J. V. G. A. Durnin and M. M. Rahaman, *Brit. J. Nutr.*, **21**, 681 (1967).

8. U. Saffiotti, R. Montesano, A. R. Sellankumar, and S. A. Borg, *Cancer*, **20**, 857 (1967).

9. M. V. Cone and P. Nettesheim, *J. Natl. Cancer Inst.*, **50**, 1599 (1973).

10. T. K. Basu, D. Donaldson, M. Jenner, D. C. Williams, and A. Sakula, *Brit. J. Cancer*, **33**, 119 (1976).

11. B. K. S. Dijkstra, *J. Natl. Cancer Inst.*, **31**, 511 (1963).

12. A. Sakula, *Brit. Med. J.*, **i**, 298 (1976).

13. V. M. Genta, D. G. Kaufman, C. C. Harris, J. M. Smith, M. B. Sporn, and U. Saffiotti, *Nature* (London), **247**, 48 (1974).

14. T. K. Basu, J. W. T. Dickerson, R. W. Raven, and D. C. Williams, *Intl. J. Vit. Nutr. Res.*, **44**, 53 (1974).

15. G. Bounous, J. M. Gentile, and J. Hugon, *Can. J. Surg.*, **14**, 312 (1971).

16. T. K. Basu and J. W. T. Dickerson, *Oncology*. In press.

17. E. M. Baker, *Am. J. Clin. Nutr.*, **20**, 583 (1967).

18. N. Krasner and I. W. Dymock, *Brit. J. Cancer*, **30**, 142 (1974).

19. T. K. Basu, R. W. Raven, J. W. T. Dickerson, and D. C. Williams, *Eur. J. Cancer*, **10**, 507 (1974).

20. A. Cushieri, *Brit. J. Surg.*, **60**, 800 (1973).

21. A. C. W. Windsor and C. B. Williams, *Brit. Med. J.*, **i**, 732 (1970).

22. G. R. Martin, S. E. Mergenhagen, and D. J. Prockop, *Nature* (London), **191**, 1008, (1961).

23. J. Gross, *J. Exp. Med.*, **109**, 557 (1959).

24. E. Cameron and A. Campbell, *Chem.-Biol., Interactions*, **9**, 285 (1974).

25. W. B. Malarkey, L. S. Jacobs, and W. H. Daughaday, *N. Engl. J. Med.*, **285**, 1160 (1971).

26. D. L. Kleinberg, G. L. Noel, and A. G. Frantz, *J. Clin. Endocrinol. Metab.*, **33**, 873 (1971).

27. M. Smethurst, T. K. Basu, and D. C. Williams, *Eur. J. Cancer*, **11**, 751 (1975).

28. H. L. Davis, R. R. Brown, J. Leklem, and I. H. Carson, *Cancer*, **31**, 1061 (1973).

29. T. K. Basu, R. W. Raven, C. Bates, and D. C. Williams, *Eur. J. Cancer*, **9**, 527 (1973).

8

Protein-losing Enteropathy in Malignancy

THOMAS A. WALDMANN, SAMUEL BRODER, AND WARREN STROBER

Metabolism Branch, National Cancer Institute, National Institutes of Health, Bethesda, Maryland

Hypoalbuminemia is an exceedingly common accompaniment of malignancy. Over 80% of patients with cancer in the large series studied by Mider and co-workers (1), Steinfeld (2), and Mariani and co-workers (3) had a reduced serum albumin concentration. In these studies the mean serum albumin concentration of the cancer patients was 2.9 g/100 ml whereas the mean albumin concentration in normal adults was 4.0 g/100 ml. The albumin concentration was lower in those patients with widespread carcinomas than in those with localized disease. In addition, there was a progressive decline in serum albumin concentration as the patient's disease progressed. Initially, decreased albumin synthesis was viewed as the sole cause for the hypoalbuminemia. Indeed, subsequent metabolic turnover studies with radioiodinated albumin have supported the conclusion that decreased albumin synthesis is the major pathophysiological mechanism responsible for the hypoalbuminemia (2, 4). Dilution of albumin in an expanded plasma volume or abnormalities of albumin distribution between the intravascular and extravascular spaces have also been contributory factors to the observed hypoalbuminemia of some patients (4). More recently, new metabolic turnover techniques have been used to demonstrate that excessive loss of serum protein into the gastrointestinal tract (protein-losing enteropathy) may also be an important factor leading to the hypoalbuminemia of many patients with neoplasia (5–9). The study of gastrointestinal protein loss in these patients is of significance in a number of ways. It provides a better understanding of the pathogenesis of the hypoalbuminemia seen in association with cancer. In addition, the use of techniques for demonstrating gastrointestinal protein loss may aid in the diagnosis of cancer, since certain patients have hypoproteinemia, edema, and gastrointestinal protein loss as the first clinical manifestations of their neoplasia. Finally, the demonstration that patients with protein-losing enteropathy due to disorders of lymphatic channel have lymphocytopenia and disorders of cell-mediated immunity provides a new insight into the pathogenesis of the immunodeficiency associated with cancer. In this chapter we shall discuss techniques for detection of protein-losing gastroenteropathy, describe the types of malignancy associated with protein-losing enteropathy, and discuss the consequences of the loss of proteins and other elements into the gastrointestinal tract. Finally, we will consider the therapy, including diet therapy, of protein-losing enteropathy in malignancy.

TECHNIQUES FOR DEMONSTRATING PROTEIN-LOSING ENTEROPATHY

All successful methods for the measurement of protein-losing enteropathy have been performed by determining the fecal excretion of radioactive labels following the intravenous administration of radiolabeled macromolecules. The radioiodinated serum proteins were the first widely used radioactive macromolecules for the study of patients with gastrointestinal protein loss. To perform a radioiodinated protein turnover, the iodinated purified protein is administered intravenously to a patient who is receiving oral iodide to block the thyroidal uptake of the isotope. Following catabolism of the labeled protein virtually all radioactivity is excreted in the urine and none is reincorporated into serum proteins. The radiolabeled protein that remains in the serum following intravenous administration is determined over the subsequent two to three weeks. In some studies the time course of decline of radioactivity in the whole body is also determined. The exact techniques used and the assumptions inherent in the various methods of analysis of iodinated protein turnover have recently been reviewed (10, 11). Serum data alone or the serum data in conjunction with whole body radioactivity data can be used to determine the total circulating albumin pool, the total exchangeable albumin pool, the rate of albumin survival or catabolism expressed either as a T½ of survival or as the fractional catabolic rate (fraction of the intravascular pool of protein catabolized per day), and the absolute catabolic rate, that is, milligrams of albumin catabolized per day. For the patient in a steady state (in whom there is no net change in the size of the body protein pools during the period of study), the absolute catabolic rate is equal to the synthetic rate.

Patients with protein-losing enteropathy associated with cancer have reduced circulating pools of albumin. The rate of albumin synthesis in these patients may be reduced, normal, or slightly increased. The survival of these proteins, however, is markedly reduced and the fractional disappearance rate (including endogenous catabolism and loss into the gastrointestinal tract) is markedly increased. The presence of a short albumin survival and an increased fractional catabolic rate for this protein suggests the possibility that protein-losing enteropathy is present. However, the occurrence of this abnormality in a given patient is still not proven, inasmuch as hypercatabolism as revealed by the turnover studies could result from an increase in the endogenous catabolic pathways without protein-losing enteropathy. Furthermore, iodine-labeled proteins cannot be used to quantitate loss of proteins into the intestinal tract because there is not only secretion of unbound radioiodide (formed upon endogenous breakdown of radiolabeled protein) into the salivary and gastric fluids but also rapid absorption of radioiodide released from proteins lost through the gastrointestinal lumen. Thus, although metabolic studies with iodinated proteins are useful in the evaluation of protein-losing enteropathy, they are not in themselves sufficient to pinpoint its presence or quantitate its magnitude.

To circumvent the limitations inherent in the use of iodinated serum proteins with respect to the measurement of protein-losing enteropathy a number of other labeled macromolecules have been introduced. These macromolecules are similar in that in each case the radioactive label is neither absorbed from the gastrointestinal lumen upon loss into the gastrointestinal tract nor excreted into the gastrointestinal lumen upon release of the label as a result of protein catabolism at a nongastrointestinal site. This characteristic of the label ensures that the label found in the stool, following intravenous administration, is an accurate representation of protein lost into gastrointestinal lumen. To quantitate protein-losing gastroenteropathy ^{51}Cr-labeled serum proteins (8, 12), ^{131}I, polyvinylpyrrolidone (13), ^{95}Nb albumin (14), ^{59}Fe dextran (15), and ^{67}Cu ceruloplasmin (16) have been utilized.

The most widely used of the radiolabeled macromolecules suitable for the quantitation of protein-losing enteropathy is ^{51}Cr-labeled albumin. We have shown that ^{51}Cr-labeled albumin is not significantly absorbed from nor secreted into the intestinal tract and that from 93 to 100% of the radioactivity of an orally administered dose of ^{51}Cr albumin appears in the subsequent fecal collections (8). Similarly, the chromium label is not secreted into the gastrointestinal tract. Thus, this material is useful for the quantitation of protein excretion into the gastrointestinal tract. In practical terms 25 μCi of ^{51}Cr albumin are administered intravenously and the subsequent fecal collection of label is measured. In the simple screening test for protein-losing enteropathy, the stools are collected free of urine in 24-hr lots for the four days after administration of the label. The stools are brought to a constant volume with water, homogenized, and counted with an appropriate standard in a gamma-ray spectrometer. The results are expressed as the percentage of the injected dose of radioactivity that is excreted in the stools during the four days after intravenous administration of the isotope. In studies of control individuals it was found that from 0 to 0.7% of the administered dose was excreted in the stools during this period, whereas patients with excessive gastrointestinal protein loss excreted significantly higher quantities of this isotope. In more sophisticated studies, the clearance of ^{51}Cr albumin expressed as a fraction of the plasma pool or as milliliters of plasma lost into the gastrointestinal tract per day is also determined. This is accomplished by relating the fecal excretion of ^{51}Cr to the serum radioactivity in a manner comparable to that used in renal clearance studies or in the study of gastrointestinal red cell loss with ^{51}Cr-labeled red cells. Normal individuals clear the protein from 5 to 35 ml of plasma per day (0.6 to 1.6% of the plasma pool daily) (8). It should be noted that there is elution of the ^{51}Cr label from the ^{51}Cr albumin molecule; thus ^{51}Cr albumin cannot be used to obtain accurate measurement of albumin synthesis and catabolism. To obtain a complete analysis of protein metabolism a combination of ^{125}I albumin and ^{51}Cr albumin turnover studies is performed. The rate of protein lost into the gastrointestinal tract is quantitated with the ^{51}Cr albumin data whereas the estimates of pool size, protein synthetic rate, and fractional catabolic rate are obtained from the ^{125}I albumin turnover data.

TYPES OF MALIGNANCIES ASSOCIATED WITH PROTEIN-LOSING ENTEROPATHY

With the use of ^{51}Cr albumin excretion studies, protein-losing enteropathy has been demonstrated in association with a wide variety of malignancies including primary tumors of the gastrointestinal tract in addition to widely disseminated neoplasms of nongastrointestinal tract origin (Table 1). In some of these patients, for example those with pancreatic carcinoma, carcinoma of the bronchus with hyponatremia, or

Table 1   Protein-losing Enteropathy with Tumors

	References
Mechanism of loss not defined	
Pancreatic carcinoma	(17)
Carcinoma of bronchus with hyponatremia or with gynecomastia	(18)
Gastric polyp	(19)
Diffuse colonic polyposis	(20,21)
Cronkhite-Canada syndrome (diffuse gastrointestinal polyps with ectodermal changes)	(22-25)
Sjögren's syndrome with reticulum cell sarcoma	(9)
Ovarian malignancy with abdominal irradiation	(9)
Multiple myeloma with amyloid deposits of bowel	(9)
Thymoma and hypogammaglobulinemia	(9)
Wiskott-Aldrich syndrome with reticulum cell sarcoma	(9)
Ulceration of the gastrointestinal mucosa	
Esophageal carcinoma	(6)
Gastric carcinoma	(6,17,26,27)
Colonic carcinoma	(6,28)
Carcinoid syndrome	(8)
Malignant melanoma metastatic to bowel	(29)
Disorders of lymphatic channels	
Lymphosarcoma or Hodgkin's disease	(17,30-35)
Mesenchymoma of mesentary	(36)
Congestive heart failure associated with carcinoid syndrome or with lymphosarcoma of chest with radiotherapy	(8) (8)

neoplasms associated with the primary immunodeficiency states, the mechanism of loss has not been defined. In others, ulceration of the gastrointestinal mucosa with loss of proteins from the mucosal surface is the primary mechanism, whereas in another group disorders of lymphatic channels are the primary defects. Excessive loss of serum proteins into the gastrointestinal tract was demonstrated in each of the seven patients with a gastric carcinoma and hypoalbuminemia that we studied (9). A four-day fecal excretion of ^{51}Cr after intravenous administration of ^{51}Cr albumin ranged from 1.1 to 7.2% of the injected dose in the patients with gastric cancer we studied as compared to a mean of 0.24% and a range of from 0.0 to 0.7% in controls. Protein-losing gastroenteropathy was also a common accompaniment of the carcinoid syndrome. Eight of the nine patients with this syndrome and hypoalbuminemia examined had protein-losing enteropathy (3). Each of the patients with the carcinoid syndrome and enteric protein loss had either an unresected primary tumor of the bowel or right heart failure. Although the majority of patients with malignant lymphoma had decreased albumin synthesis as the sole cause of their hypoalbuminemia (4), a significant subset of these patients was identified who had excessive gastrointestinal protein loss. For example, we have identified six patients with a malignant lymphoma who had increased four-day fecal ^{51}Cr albumin excretion rates that ranged from 1 to 10.4% of the injected dose (9). Two of these patients with lymphoma and hypoalbuminemia had protein clearance rates of 385 and 420 ml of plasma into the gastrointestinal tract per day as compared to the normal clearance range of 5 to 35 ml per day. These studies established that enteric protein loss is a major factor in the hypoalbuminemia of some patients with lymphoma. It is clear from our studies and also those of others that protein-losing enteropathy represents a significant factor in the hypoproteinemia of a wide variety of neoplastic diseases. In many of the patients with neoplastic diseases, an increase in the rate of enteric protein loss is only one of several abnormalities, and the primary malignant disease is readily apparent from other more prominent signs and symptoms. In contrast, in some patients, unexplained edema and hypoproteinemia are the presenting symptoms; in these patients, the demonstration of protein-losing enteropathy was the initial clue to the detection of a potentially fatal but treatable disorder.

MECHANISMS OF PROTEIN-LOSING ENTEROPATHY IN MALIGNANCY

Inflammation and ulceration of a region of the mucosa of the gastrointestinal tract with loss of exudate that contains plasma proteins would appear to be a pathophysiological mechanism that explains the excessive gastrointestinal protein loss in patients with esophageal, gastric, and colonic carcinomas, and is also a contributing factor in patients with ulcerating carcinoid tumors of the stomach and small bowel. In addition, the patients with metastases that involve the small intestine may also have excessive enteric protein loss by a similar mechanism. A second major cause of protein-losing enteropathy that appears to be of significance in some patients with malignant lymphoma, in patients with mesenteric mesenchymoma, as well as in some patients with neoplasms and congestive heart failure is a disorder of intestinal lymphatic channels. This disorder of intestinal lymphatics leads to the loss of proteins, minerals such as calcium, iron, and copper, as well as lymphocytes into the gastrointestinal lumen. That such a disorder of intestinal lymphatic channels is of significance in the protein-losing enteropathy of some of these patients is suggested by certain data. First, four of the six patients we studied with lymphoma and protein-losing enteropathy had chylous effusions. Second, markedly dilated lymphatic channels of the small intestinal villi have been demonstrated in some of these patients on gastrointestinal biopsy. Finally, all of the patients had lymphocytopenia, a feature that is noted in association with all forms of protein-losing enteropathy due to lymphatic abnormalities (37–39).

The disorders of intestinal lymphatic channels in patients with malignant disease may be due to neoplastic obstruction of central and mesenteric lymph nodes and lymphatic channels. Alternatively, patients may have cardiac disease with right heart failure and an increased central venous pressure that results in increased lymph production and increased thoracic duct pressure with a functional obstruction to entry of lymph into the central veins (39–41). This is most likely in patients with endocardial fibrosis of the carcinoid syndrome or in patients with constrictive pericarditis due to tumor involvement of pericardium or due to mediastinal radiotherapy for malignancy.

PATHOPHYSIOLOGICAL AND IMMUNOLOGICAL CONSEQUENCES OF PROTEIN-LOSING ENTEROPATHY IN MALIGNANCY

There are many consequences of protein-losing enteropathy in patients with malignancy. In all of the groups of patients with malignancy and protein-losing enteropathy, there is a reduction in the serum concentration of the long-surviving serum proteins, such as albumin. At the initiation of protein-losing enteropathy there is a marked increase in the fractional and absolute disappearance rate of albumin. This is due, in large measure, to loss of this protein into the gastrointestinal tract. The proteins lost into the gastrointestinal tract are catabolized to their constituent amino acids, which are reabsorbed. However, the absolute synthetic rate for albumin remains normal or only modestly increased since the body's capacity to increase albumin synthesis is very limited. Thus, since the absolute disappearance rate is greater than the synthetic rate, there is a progressive decrease in the albumin pool size until the product of the elevated fractional catabolic rate and the reduced total circulating albumin pool size is again equal to the absolute synthetic rate for albumin. Thus, a new steady state is achieved in patients with protein-losing enteropathy with a reduced serum albumin concentration due primarily to the short survival of this protein. Because of the hypo-proteinemia, the patients accumulate edema fluid.

As noted above, there are a number of patients with protein-losing gastroenteropathy secondary to disorders of lymphatic channels. The edema accumulation in these patients may be asymmetrical and may be associated with the development of chylous effusions. Those patients with protein-losing enteropathy associated with lymphatic abnormalities have severe immunological consequences due to the loss of lymphocytes into the gastrointestinal tract. These patients have what is in effect a fistula between the thoracic duct and their gastrointestinal tract with loss of the population of lymphocytes that normally circulates into the central lymphatic channels. As a consequence, these individuals have lymphocytopenia and an immune deficiency state characterized by an abnormality of cell-mediated immunity. Such patients are similar to those with benign conditions associated with abnormal lymphatic channels, such as intestinal lymphangiectasia, Whipple's disease, and congestive heart failure associated with protein-losing enteropathy with lymphocytopenia (9, 38, 39). Thus, the mean lymphocyte count of the patients with lymphosarcoma and protein-losing enteropathy and disorders of lymphatic channels was $350\pm 100/mm^3$ as compared with $2500\pm 600/mm^3$ in a control group of individuals (9). In vitro studies of lymphocyte function have shown that in patients with disorders of lymphatic channels the population of lymphocytes that are necessary for cell-mediated immunity is relatively depleted; that is, lymphocytes of patients with such disorders have impaired in vitro transformation to nonspecific mitogens, to specific antigens, and to allogeneic cells when compared to equal numbers of lymphocytes from normal individuals (37, 38). As a consequence of their lymphocytopenia and preferential depletion in long-lived recirculating lymphocytes, both patients with lymphosarcoma and other tumors associated with disorders of lymphatic channels and patients with intestinal lymphangiectasia have abnormalities of cell-mediated immunity. These patients are unable to manifest positive skin test reactions to such common antigens as mumps, *Trichophyton, Candida albicans*, streptokinase-streptodornase, tetanus, or diphtheria, whereas over 97% of normal controls have positive responses to one or more of these agents (38). In addition, these patients cannot be sensitized with dinitrochlorobenzene, whereas over 95% of the control population can be sensitized with this agent. In addition, these individuals cannot reject skin grafts from unrelated individuals.

This decrease in cell-mediated immune function in patients with neoplasms and lymphocytopenia due to lymphatic obstruction and loss of lymphocytes into the gastrointestinal tract predisposes such patients to infections with fungal agents and low-grade pathogens. This process could also further weaken the immunological surveillance defense mechanisms against the growth of the neoplasm.

THERAPY OF THE PROTEIN-LOSING ENTEROPATHY ASSOCIATED WITH MALIGNANCY

The most valuable technique for the reversal of the protein and lymphocyte loss into the gastrointestinal tract associated with malignancy is the effective therapy of the tumor. There has been a complete reversal of the protein-losing enteropathy after surgical removal of the carcinoma of the colon or of the stomach and of a gastric polyp with malignant changes (6, 20, 30). In addition, there was also reversal of protein-losing enteropathy after effective therapy of patients with lymphoma with chemotherapeutic agents such as chlorambucil (32, 33). In many patients, however, therapy directed against the tumor has not been effective. In those patients with protein-losing enteropathy associated with disorders of lymphatic channels a low fat diet may be of value. Thus, over half of the patients with protein-losing enteropathy associated with a disorder of lymphatic channels placed on a low fat diet had a significant increase in the blood lymphocyte numbers and serum protein concentration with a reduction of edema. Jefferies and co-workers (42) and Holt (43) have shown that albumin survival returns toward normal following institution of a low fat diet or a diet that had middle chain triglycerides replacing long chain triglycerides. The use of a low fat diet or a diet using middle chain triglycerides which are absorbed into the portal vein rather than through the intestinal lymphatics would be expected to have its effect by a reduction of lymph flow and pressure in these patients with disordered lymphatic function.

SUMMARY

Metabolic studies with radioiodinated albumin have led to the conclusion that decreased albumin synthesis is the major pathophysiological mechanism responsible for the hypoalbuminemia that very often accompanies malignancy. Studies with ^{51}Cr albumin have shown, however, that excessive loss of proteins into the gastrointestinal tract is also an important factor in the cause of the hypoalbuminemia in many patients with neoplasia. Protein-losing enteropathy due to ulceration of a region of mucosa of the gastrointestinal tract, with loss of exudate that contains plasma proteins, was demonstrated in patients with carcinoma of the esophagus, stomach, and colon and in patients with unresected gastrointestinal carcinoid tumors. A second major cause of protein-losing enteropathy, a disorder of intestinal lymphatic channels with loss of protein and lymphocyte-rich lymph into the gastrointestinal tract, was observed in patients with lymphosarcoma and Hodgkin's disease and in patients with congestive heart failure associated with the carcinoid syndrome or constrictive pericarditis. All of the patients with protein-losing enteropathy associated with malignancy develop hypoproteinemia, and in many cases edema. Patients with protein-losing enteropathy due to disorders of lymphatic channels have, in addition, lymphocytopenia, inability to manifest delayed hypersensitivity skin reactions, and inability to reject skin grafts due to the loss of lymphocytes into the gastrointestinal tract. These patients have an increased incidence of infections with fungal agents and have a decrease in their immunological surveillance defense mechanisms against their tumors. The most valuable technique for the therapy of protein-losing enteropathy associated with malignancy is surgical, radiotherapeutic, or chemotherapeutic treatment of the tumor itself. However, in those patients with protein-losing enteropathy associated with disordered lymphatic channels the use of a low fat diet or a diet in which long chain triglycerides are replaced by middle chain triglycerides may lead to a significant increase in the circulating protein and lymphocyte levels and to a diminution in the edema and the disorders of cell-mediated immunity.

REFERENCES

1. G. B. Mider, E. L. Alling, and J. J. Morton, *Cancer,* **3**, 56 (1950).

2. J. L. Steinfeld, *Cancer,* **13**, 974 (1960).

3. G. Mariani, W. Strober, H. Keiser, and T. A. Waldmann. *Cancer,* **38**, 854 (1976).

4. T. Waldmann, J. Trier, and H. Fallon, *J. Clin. Invest.* **42**, 171 (1963).

5. S. Jarnum and M. Schwartz, *Gastroenterology* **38**, 769 (1960).

6. P. T. Sum, M. M. Hoffman, and D. R. Webster, *Can. J. Surg.,* **7**, 1 (1964).

7. S. von Barandun, J. Aebersold, R. Bianchi, R. Kluthe, G. von Muralt, G. Poretti, and G. Riva, *Schweiz. Med. Wochschr.,* **90**, 1458 (1960).

8. T. A. Waldmann, R. D. Wochner, and W. Strober, *Am. J. Med.,* **46**, 275 (1969).

9. T. A. Waldmann, S. Broder, and W. Strober, *Ann. N.Y. Acad. Sci.,* **230**, 306 (1974).

10. L. Donato, C. M. E. Matthews, B. Nosslin, G. Segre, and F. Vitek, *J. Nucl. Biol. Med.,* **10**, 3 (1966).

11. T. A. Waldmann and W. Strober, *Progr. Allergy* **13**, 1 (1969).

12. T. A. Waldmann, *Lancet* **2**, 121 (1961).

13. R. S. Gordon, Jr., *Lancet,* **1**, 325 (1959).

14. K. N. Jeejeebhoy, S. Jarnum, B. Singh, G. D. Nadkarni, and H. Westergaard, *Scand. J. Gastroenterol.,* **3**, 449 (1968).

15. S. B. Andersen and S. Jarnum, *Lancet,* **1**, 1060 (1966).

16. T. A. Waldmann, A. G. Morell, R. D. Wochner, W. Strober, and I. Sternlieb, *J. Clin. Invest.,* **46**, 10 (1967).

17. P. Bernades, M. Lewin, and S. Bonfils, *Rev. Eur. Etud. Clin. Biol.,* **16**, 887 (1971).

18. A. M. Dawson, R. Williams, and H. S. Williams, *Brit. Med. J.,* **2**, 667 (1961).

19. J. Dich, H. Paaby, and M. Schwartz, *Brit. Med. J.* **2**, 686 (1969).

20. A. Wagner and W. Wenz, *Schweiz. Med. Wochschr.,* **99**, 777 (1969).

21. V. Varro, G. Baradnay, L. Csernay, and E. Sovenyi, *Orv. Hetilap.,* **109**, 83 (1968).

22. G. A. von Martini and W. Dolle, *Deutsch. Med. Wochschr.,* **86**, 2524 (1961).

23. S. Jarnum and H. Jensen, *Gastroenterology,* **50**, 107 (1966).

24. H. Orimo, T. Fujita, M. Yoshikawa, T. Takemoto, Y. Matsuo, and K. Nakao, *Am. J. Med.,* **47**, 445 (1969).

25. J. Takahata, K. Okubo, T. Komeda, T. Kono, and I. Fukui, *Digestion,* **5**, 153 (1972).

26. G. B. J. Glass and A. Ishimori, *Am. J. Digest. Dis.* [*N.S.*], **16**, 103 (1961).

27. J. Wetterfors, S. O. Liljeddahl, L. O. Plaintin, and G. Birke, *Acta Med. Scand.,* **172**, 163 (1962).

28. L. S. Valberg, S. N. Huang, and J. Ludwig, *Can. Med. Assn. J.,* **98**, 638 (1968).

29. H. Goebell, H. Dombrowski, P. Schmitz-Moormann, and G. A. Martini, *Internist,* **11**, 142 (1970).

30. M. Schwartz and S. Jarnum, *Danish Med. Bull.,* **8**, 1 (1961).

31. H. Bennhold and H. Ott, *Med. Klin.,* **57**, 814 (1962).

32. D. Werdegar, H. Alder, and C. Watlington, *Ann. Intern. Med.,* **59**, 207 (1963).

33. H. Pequignot, J. Guerre, J. Debray, B. Christoforov, P. Van Amerongen, and J. J. Cocheton, *Semaine Hop. Paris,* **45**, 1758 (1969).

34. J. Vague, J. L. Codaccioni, J. F. Delmont, Y. Ayme, J. Nicolino, J. Grisoli, and H. Payan, *Marseille Med.,* **100**, 77 (1963).

35. G. Marenco, R. Rembado P. Cavaliere, and P. Biscaldi, *Pathologica,* **61**, 463 (1969).

36. L. A. Rosati and H. A. Oberman, *Arch. Intern. Med.,* **122**, 50 (1968).

37. T. A. Waldmann, *Gastroenterology,* **50**, 422 (1966).

38. W. Strober, R. D. Wochner, P. P. Carbone, and T. A. Waldmann, *J. Clin. Invest.,* **46**, 1643 (1967).

39. W. Strober, L. S. Cohen, T. A. Waldmann, and E. Braunwald, *Am. J. Med.,* **44**, 842 (1968).

40. J. D. Davidson, T. A. Waldmann, D. S. Goodman, and R. S. Gordon, Jr., *Lancet,* **1**, 899 (1961).

41. V. P. Petersen and P. Ottosen, *Acta Med. Scand.,* **176**, 335 (1964).

42. G. H. Jeffries, A. Chapman, and M. H. Sleisenger, *N. Engl. J. Med.,* **270**, 761 (1964).

43. P. Holt, *Pediatrics,* **34**, 629 (1964).

Prevention and Therapy

9

Vitamin A and its Analogs (Retinoids) in Cancer Prevention

MICHAEL B. SPORN

National Cancer Institute, Bethesda, Maryland

The chronicity of the process of the development of malignant disease of epithelia makes a preventive approach to cancer an attractive possibility. It is well established that the development of invasive cancer of epithelia of the lung, bladder, breast, uterine cervix, and other important target sites is a prolonged process that may take up to 20 years or more in man before reaching its terminal invasive stage (1). The phenomena of tumor progression and tumor promotion have been studied at length (2,3), and by now it is well established that the pathogenesis of most epithelial cancers involves a prolonged series of premalignant cytological changes before clones of malignant cells, which have the capacity for invasion and metastasis, are produced.

During premalignant stages of epithelial disease, the pathogenesis of epithelial cancer is potentially arrestable or reversible by intrinsic physiological controls (4). Indeed, were it not for these intrinsic controls, the incidence of invasive cancer in man would be much higher than the present figures, which are already of great distress. The study of intrinsic physiologic controls in epithelia, which prevent the development of clones of malignant cells, and the development of pharmacological methods to enhance these protective mechanisms, is a topic of great importance for cancer research at present. The conventional cytotoxic approach to cancer chemotherapy, in which a deliberate attempt is made to kill cancer cells by selectively blocking DNA, RNA, or protein synthesis or other key metabolic pathways in the cancer cell, has not been strikingly successful for treatment of invasive epithelial cancers, such as those of the lung, bladder, breast, and uterine cervix (5). As an alternative to this approach of cytotoxic chemotherapy, we have suggested the development of a new pharmacological approach to prevention of cancer, which we have called "chemoprevention" (6,7). This alternative approach relies on pharmacological enhancement of intrinsic physiological mechanisms that exist in epithelia to arrest or prevent the development of malignant cells. This approach does not require the use of cytotoxic agents. However, in order to be effective, chemoprevention must be applied during premalignant stages of disease. Once invasive malignancy has resulted, the traditional modalities of surgery, radiation, and cytotoxic chemotherapy still are the only means at hand for effective arrest or cure of malignancy. In the remainder of this chapter, recent progress in the use of vitamin A and its synthetic analogs (together called retinoids) for chemoprevention of cancer will be summarized.

IMPORTANCE OF RETINOIDS FOR EPITHELIAL DIFFERENTIATION

It is well known that retinoids are required for normal cellular differentiation of most, if not all, epithelia which account for the great majority of all cancer in men and women (Table 1). These epithelia include those of the bronchi and trachea, stomach, intestine, uterus, kidney and bladder, testis, prostate, pancreatic ducts, breast, and skin (9). The retinoids act to control normal cell differentiation in these epithelial target sites in a manner that resembles the control of uterine cell differentiation by estrogenic hormones or prostatic cell differentiation by androgenic hormones. The main difference is that the mammalian body does not have the capacity for synthesis of retinoids, in contrast to its intrinsic ability to synthesize steroids. If retinoids are not present in the diet, mature differentiated cells, such as ciliated and mucus cells of the bronchial epithelium, transitional cells of the bladder epithelium, or ductular epithelial cells of the pancreas and salivary glands, are no longer formed from the underlying epithelial basal cells (10). Instead, an alternative pathway of differentiation is followed, leading to the formation of keratinizing squamous cells, which eventually replace the normal mature epithelial cells. This process of squamous metaplasia caused by retinoid deficiency is reversible, however. Administration of retinoids will reverse the formation of keratinizing squamous cells and cause reappearance of the appropriate mature differentiated cells.

In addition to their ability to control normal cell differentiation in target epithelia, retinoids are also capable of reversing premalignant cellular changes caused in target epithelia by chemical carcinogens. This

Table 1   Retinoid Dependency of Epithelium from Principal Sites of Cancer in Man

Site and Number of Estimated Cancer Deaths USA, 1975 (8)[a]		Retinoid Dependency of Normal Epithelium
Lung	81,000	Yes
Colon-rectum	49,000	Yes
Bone marrow and lymph nodes	34,000	Nonepithelial malignancy
Breast	33,000	Yes
Pancreas	20,000	Yes
Prostate	19,000	Yes
Stomach	14,000	Yes
Ovary	11,000	???
Liver	10,000	Yes (bile ducts only)
Bladder	9,000	Yes
Total	280,000	

[a] Total estimated cancer deaths, USA, 1975: 365,000.

has been studied most extensively in organ cultures of mouse prostate, in which premalignant cellular changes can be induced by chemical carcinogens. After lesions have been formed in these prostatic organ cultures by the carcinogens, application of retinoids will cause a reversal of the premalignant changes and the reappearance of new epithelial cells which have a normal morphology (11–14). Similar results have recently been obtained with organ cultures of tracheal epithelium (15). All of these findings indicate a fundamental role for retinoids in control of the process of cellular differentiation, both normal and premalignant, in target epithelia. The application of these basic considerations to prevention of invasive malignancy in the intact animal will now be considered.

PREVENTION OF EPITHELIAL CANCER BY RETINOIDS

Early attempts to use retinoids for cancer prevention in animals involved the use of natural retinoids, such as the vitamin A esters retinyl palmitate and retinyl acetate, since these were the only retinoids available for studies at the time. A review of this earlier literature has recently been published (6), and we will not attempt a complete summary. Suffice it to say that conclusions reached are often conflicting, although on closer inspection one finds that rarely have two separate groups of investigators repeated identical experimental protocols. It is clear, at present, that natural retinoids such as retinyl esters are of restricted usefulness for cancer prevention because of two major limitations:

1. Natural retinoids such as retinyl esters may not reach the desired epithelial target sites in sufficient quantity because of special mechanisms for transport of retinol and storage of retinyl esters in the liver.
2. Natural retinoids such as retinyl esters have a high potential for toxicity if they are fed chronically in high doses, because of the excessive storage of these compounds in the liver.

Thus, although early studies indicated that retinyl esters might be of use in prevention of carcinoma of the stomach (16), vagina (16), uterine cervix (16), trachea (17), and bronchus (17), conflicting results were obtained by other investigators. In all experiments performed with retinyl esters, problems of toxicity or achieving adequate tissue distribution were always encountered. These problems led to investigation of other retinoids, which would have different pharmacokinetic and toxicologic properties. The first such retinoid to be investigated was all-*trans*-retinoic acid, which Bollag showed to be effective in prevention of skin carcinomas induced by the polycyclic hydrocarbon 7,12-dimethylbenz(*a*)anthracene, and croton oil (18). In contrast to retinol or retinyl esters, retinoic acid is not transported in the blood by retinol binding protein, but rather by serum albumin (19). Moreover, chronic feeding of retinoic acid does not lead to deposition of retinoid in the liver (20). Thus, the pattern of tissue distribution and storage of retinoic acid is very different from the pattern that holds for retinyl esters. However, retinoic acid is not without its own undesirable toxic side effects, particularly because of its ability to damage lysosomal membranes, and its practical usefulness in cancer prevention is limited by this toxicity (21).

Because of the above considerations, a vigorous search has begun to find new synthetic retinoids that would have the desired pharmacological properties for prevention of epithelial cancer, and be relatively free of the toxic properties that had previously limited the effective use of these agents. At present, data are available which show that synthetic retinoids, in which the ring, side chain, or polar terminal group of the retinoid molecule has been modified, may be used to prevent carcinoma of the skin (22,23), tracheobronchial epithelium (24), mammary gland (25), and bladder (26).

The first successful use of synthetic retinoids in prevention of epithelial cancer was by Bollag, who showed that two retinoids, containing an aromatic ring (Fig. 1b), rather than a cyclohexenyl ring (Fig. 1a), were effective in prevention of skin papillomas and carcinomas in mice (22,23). In addition to alteration of the ring, the compounds used by Bollag had synthetic alteration of the terminal group; compounds with either a carboxylic acid ethyl ester (22) or a carboxylic acid ethyl amide (23) terminal group were used in his experiments.

Another synthetic retinoid that has been used in several studies is 13-*cis*-retinoic acid. This analog is much less toxic than all-*trans*-retinoic acid and may be fed chronically without harm to rats or hamsters at relatively high dose levels (27). The first use of 13-*cis*-retinoic acid in prevention of cancer in an experimental animal was by Port, Kaufman, and Sporn, who used this agent to inhibit the development of respiratory cancer induced in hamsters by intratracheal administration of benzo(*a*)pyrene–ferric oxide mixtures (24). Lifetime oral administration of 9 milligrams of 13-*cis*-retinoic acid per week resulted in no evident toxicity to the hamsters and significantly depressed the incidence of respiratory squamous carcinoma caused by the benzo(*a*)pyrene–ferric oxide mixture. Based on these results, it was decided to investigate the effects of 13-*cis*-retinoic acid in prevention of bladder cancer in the rat, since the pathogenesis of respiratory cancer and bladder cancer have many similar features. It had already been shown that feeding of retinyl palmitate was ineffective in protecting the rat from bladder cancer induced by a potent nitrofuran carcinogen (28), and a more polar retinoid, such as 13-*cis*-retinoic acid, which would have better pharmacokinetic properties, was desired for these experiments. The new experimental system developed by Hicks and Wakefield (29) for induction of bladder cancer in the rat was used for these experiments with 13-*cis*-retinoic acid. Rats were given three biweekly doses of the carcinogen N-methyl-N-nitrosourea by direct instillation into the urinary bladder.

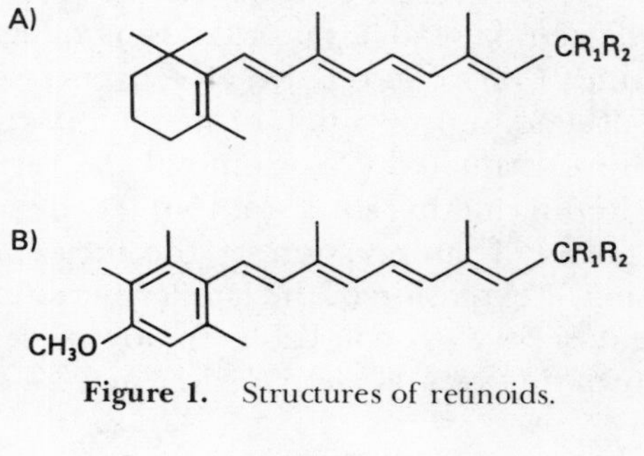

Figure 1.   Structures of retinoids.

After completion of dosing with this direct-acting carcinogen, which requires no metabolic activation, the rats were divided into several groups, which were treated with either no retinoid, or 13-*cis*-retinoic acid at a low dose (120 mg per kilo of diet), or a high dose (300 mg per kilo of diet). The retinoid was incorporated into the diet of the animals and fed for eight months, at which time all animals were killed. A thorough histological examination of the bladder epithelium was then performed and the incidence and extent of neoplasia was determined on a series of randomized and coded slides. It was found that feeding of 13-*cis*-retinoic acid at the high dose caused a marked diminution in the number of rats with bladder neoplasms, as well as in the extent of neoplasia within the bladders (26). Particularly striking was the effect of the retinoid in diminishing the presence and extent both of flat, proliferative lesions, which had varying degrees of hypercellularity and atypia, and of squamous metaplastic lesions. These effects on both neoplastic and preneoplastic lesions clearly were not caused by some generalized toxic effect of 13-*cis*-retinoic acid. No manifestations of retinoid toxicity were seen in the rats, and the average weights of the rats fed 13-*cis*-retinoic acid were essentially the same as those of the rats fed chow diet alone.

Synthetic retinoids have also been used to prevent the development of mammary cancer in the experimental animal. It had originally been reported by Schmahl and co-workers (30) that retinyl palmitate was ineffective in preventing mammary cancer when given once a week in a large intra gastric dose following the carcinogen 7,12-dimethylbenz*(a)*-anthracene (DMBA). The use of retinyl ester to prevent mammary cancer induced by DMBA has recently been reinvestigated in a study in which retinyl acetate was fed chronically in the diet to rats, following administration of DMBA. A definite protective effect of retinyl acetate was found in these studies (31), but a synthetic retinoid with better pharmacological properties was again desired. Retinyl methyl ether was chosen because it had been shown to be less toxic than retinyl acetate (32), and because it had been shown to yield a greater concentration of retinoid in the mammary gland and adjacent fat pad, after oral dosing of equivalent doses of these two compounds (33). The relative effectiveness of retinyl methyl ether and retinyl acetate in prevention of mammary cancer induced by DMBA was therefore evaluated (25). Some of the results obtained are shown in Table 2. Retinyl methyl ether was found to be superior to retinyl acetate, both in terms of suppression of the incidence of mammary cancer, and in terms of extension of the latency period for development of cancers. At the dose levels used (Table 2), no toxic effects were seen. However, it is known that retinyl methyl ether may be cleaved to retinol

Table 2   Effects of Retinyl Acetate and Retinyl Methyl Ether on Mammary Carcinogenesis Induced by 7,12-Dimethylbenz(a)anthracene (DMBA)[a]

Group	Retinoid	Number of Rats	% Incidence of Palpable Mammary Cancers at 120 Days	% Incidence of Palpable Mammary Cancers at 180 Days	Mean No. of Mammary Cancers Per Rat at 180 Days
A	None	50	20	32	0.42
B	Retinyl acetate, 760 μmoles per kg of diet	30	12	23	0.27
C	Retinyl methyl ether, 760 μmoles per kg of diet	20	0	10	0.15

[a]Sprague-Dawley female rats, 50 days of age, were given a single oral dose of 5 mg of DMBA. One week later, two groups were started on diets containing either retinyl acetate or retinyl methyl ether, while a third group was continued on normal chow diet. Mammary tumors were palpated weekly, and all animals were killed at 180 days for histological evaluation (31).

and be stored in the liver as retinyl ester (34,35). Thus, although retinyl methyl ether is superior to retinyl acetate for suppression of experimental breast cancer, the potential storage of metabolites of this compound in the liver suggests that it may also have undesirable effects if fed for very long periods of time. The development of other retinoid ethers that would have the desirable effects on prevention of breast cancer without the potential for accumulation in the liver would thus seem to be a highly desirable goal.

METHODS FOR EVALUATING NEW RETINOIDS

It is thus already clear that the future practical use of retinoids in cancer prevention will depend on the use of synthetic retinoids. Since the evaluation of the ability of large numbers of new retinoids to prevent various types of epithelial cancer in the experimental animal is very expensive and time consuming, new methods must be developed as a screen for potential usefulness in the live animal. Several new in vitro assays, which use organ culture methods, have been developed recently for this purpose. These assays can be used to measure desired effects of retinoids on control of epithelial cell differentiation, both normal and premalignant, as well as undesirable toxic effects of retinoids.

The in vitro assay that has been used most extensively in evaluating the relationship between structure of retinoids and their ability to control normal cell differentiation employs tracheal organ cultures (33). Retinoid-deficient tracheal organ cultures undergo epithelial squamous metaplasia and keratinization, which is reversible upon addition of retinoids to the organ cultures. A large number of retinoids have been evaluated in this system (Fig. 1, Table 3). Toxic effects of retinoids on cartilage have also been evaluated in organ cultures, employing either rabbit ear cartilage (21), or hamster tracheal cartilage (33), as shown in Table 3. Dose-response curves may be plotted for both the desired effects on activity (Fig. 2) and the undesired toxic effects (Fig. 3). Some of the results that have been obtained in these assays (33) may be summarized as follows:

1. although the presence of a terminal carboxylic acid group may be associated with high activity, it also may convey a high degree of toxicity;

Table 3   Activity of Retinoids in Tracheal Organ Culture [a]

Structure, $R_1 =$, $R_2 =$	Trivial Name	Reversal of Keratinization, Tracheal Organ Culture, ED_{50}, M	Toxicity to Cartilage, Tracheal Organ Culture, TD_{20}, M
Fig. 1A, $-H_2$, $-OH$	Retinol	2×10^{-9} (54)	2×10^{-6} (67)
Fig. 1A, $-H_2$, $-OCH_3$	Retinyl methyl ether	3×10^{-9} (122)	1×10^{-5} (103)
Fig. 1A, $-H_2$, $-OC_4H_9$	Retinyl butyl ether	3×10^{-8} (55)	not toxic at 1×10^{-5} (42)
Fig. 1A, $-H_2$, $-OCOCH_3$	Retinyl acetate	3×10^{-9} (123)	6×10^{-6} (63)
Fig. 1A, $-H_2$, $-NHCOCH_3$	Retinyl N-acetyl amine	9×10^{-9} (113)	not toxic at 1×10^{-5} (50)

Table 3 *(continued)*

Structure $R_1 =$, $R_2 =$	Trivial Name	Reversal of Keratinization, Trachael Organ Culture, ED_{50}, M	Toxicity to Cartilage, Trachael Organ Culture, TD_{20}, M
Fig. 1A, $-H_2$, $-N(CO)_2C_6H_4$	Retinyl N-phthalimide	5×10^{-7} (49)	not toxic at 1×10^{-5} (10)
Fig. 1A, $-H$, $=O$	Retinal	3×10^{-10} (98)	5×10^{-7} (49)
Fig. 1A, $-H$, $=NNHCOCH_3$	Retinal acetylhydrazone	4×10^{-10} (54)	7×10^{-7} (25)
Fig 1A, $=O$, $-OH$	Retinoic acid	3×10^{-10} (337)	1×10^{-7} (116)
Fig. 1A, $=O$, $-OC_2H_5$	Retinoic acid ethyl ester	5×10^{-10} (119)	2×10^{-7} (18)
Fig. 1A, $=O$, $-NHC_2H_5$	Retinoic acid ethyl amide	2×10^{-9} (52)	9×10^{-7} (32)
Fig. 1B, $-H_2$, $-OH$	TMMP analog of retinol	2×10^{-8} (48)	9×10^{-7} (34)
Fig. 1B, $-H_2$, $-OCH_3$	TMMP analog of retinyl methyl ether	2×10^{-8} (70)	4×10^{-6} (57)
Fig. 1B, $=O$, $-OH$	TMMP analog of retinoic acid	6×10^{-9} (187)	6×10^{-8} (88)
Fig. 1B, $=O$, $-OC_2H_5$	TMMP analog of retinoic acid ethyl ester	2×10^{-8} (53)	2×10^{-7} (63)
Fig. 1B, $=O$, $-NHC_2H_5$	TMMP analog of retinoic acid ethyl amide	3×10^{-8} (66)	1×10^{-6} (52)

[a] ED_{50} (M) for reversal of keratinization in tracheal organ culture is the dose for reversal of keratinization in epithelium of 50% of retinoid-deficient hamster tracheas using standard assay conditions (33). TD_{20} (M) for toxicity to trachela organ culture is the dose for release of 20% of total proteoglycan from hamster tracheal cartilage into culture medium using standard assay conditions (33). Numbers of organ cultures used for evaluating each retinoid are shown in parentheses. Reprinted, with permission, from (33).

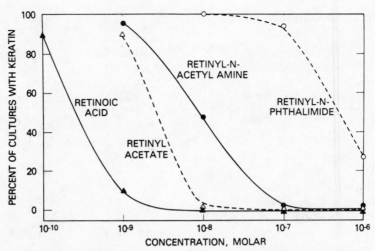

Figure 2. Dose-response curves for reversal of keratinization in organ cultures of retinoid-deficient tracheal epithelium by application of retinoids. Tracheas (one per culture dish) were treated with retinoids for four days before scoring for the presence of both keratin and keratohyaline granules. Similar curves were obtained for all retinoids reported in Table 3, and the ED_{50} was derived from these plots. Numbers of tracheas used in these experiments are shown in Table 3. Reprinted, with permission, from (33).

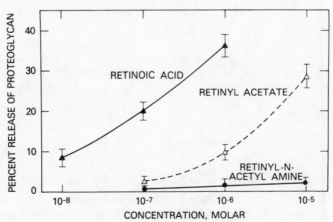

Figure 3. Dose-response curves for toxic effects of retinoids to tracheal organ culture. Tracheas (one per culture dish) were treated with retinoids for three days before measuring both proteoglycan released into the culture medium, and that remaining in the cartilage. Standard error of the mean of measurements is shown. Numbers of tracheas used in these experiments are shown in Table 3. Reprinted, with permission, from (33).

2. a terminal amine function, as in retinyl N-acetyl amine, is compatible with activity and may result in an analog with low toxicity; and
3. modification of the polar terminal group can markedly lessen toxicity without major loss of activity, as can be seen with retinal methyl ether.

Still another important type of in vitro assay is that which measures the ability of retinoids to reverse the hyperplastic and anaplastic epithelial lesions caused by chemical carcinogens in organ culture. This property of retinoids was first reported by Lasnitzki (11), using prostate organ cultures. Recent studies by Chopra and Wilkoff (12,13), as well as by Lasnitzki (14), have shown that a large number of retinoids have the direct ability to control premalignant cell differentiation in this system. The phenomenon is not limited to prostatic epithelium, since Lane and Miller have recently shown that retinoids can reverse the effects of benzo(a)pyrene on rat tracheal epithelium in organ culture (15).

CONCLUSIONS

We have summarized the data, by now quite extensive, which indicate that retinoids may be used to control both normal and premalignant cell differentiation, both in vivo and in vitro. The practical usefulness of such agents to prevent cancer in man remains to be shown. Advances still need to be made in synthesis of more active or less toxic retinoids. However, the data at hand now warrant consideration of the use of retinoids such as 13-*cis*-retinoic acid for prevention of epithelial cancer in high risk human populations.

ACKNOWLEDGMENTS

I am greatly indebted to my colleagues Drs. Charles Brown, Clinton Grubbs, Richard Moon, Robert Squire, and Martin Wenk for their many contributions to the animal studies reported here. Our collaboration with Hoffmann-La Roche Inc., Nutley, New Jersey, and F. Hoffmann-La Roche and Co., A. G., Basel, Switzerland, has afforded not only the retinoids used in these studies, but also many useful discussions with members of their staff. I also thank Nancy Dunlop, Dianne Newton, Doris Overman, and Joseph Smith for valuable technical and secretarial assistance.

REFERENCES

1. E. Farber and M. B. Sporn, Eds., Symposium "Early Lesions and the Development of Epithelial Cancer," *Cancer Res.,* **36**, 2475 (1976).

2. L. Foulds, *Neoplastic Development,* Academic Press, New York, (1969).

3. R. K. Boutwell, *CRC Crit. Rev. Toxicol.,* **2**, 419 (1974).

4. J. Cairns, *Nature,* **255**, 197 (1975).

5. E. Silverberg and A. I. Holleb, *CA,* **25**, 2 (1975).

6. M. B. Sporn, N. M. Dunlop, D. L. Newton, and J. M. Smith, *Fed. Proc.,* **35**, 1332 (1976).

7. M. B. Sporn, *Cancer Res.,* **36**, 2699 (1976).

8. National Cancer Institute, Fact Book, Bethesda, Md. (1975), p. 20.

9. T. Moore, *in* W. H. Sebrell and R. S. Harris, Eds., *The Vitamins,* 2nd Ed., Vol. 1, Academic Press, New York (1967), p. 245.

10. S. B. Wolbach and P. R. Howe, *J. Exp. Med.,* **42**, 753 (1925).

11. I. Lasnitzki, *Brit. J. Cancer,* **9**, 434 (1955).

12. D. P. Chopra and L. J. Wilkoff, *J. Natl. Cancer Inst.,* **56**, 583 (1976).

13. D. P. Chopra and L. J. Wilkoff, *J. Natl. Cancer Inst.,* in press.

14. I. Lasnitzki, *Brit. J. Cancer,* **34**, 239 (1976).

15. B. P. Lane and S. L. Miller, *Proc. Am. Assn. Cancer Res.,* **17**,211 (1976).

16. E. W. Chu and R. A. Malmgren, *Cancer Res.,* **25**, 884 (1965).

17. U. Saffiotti, R. Montesano, A. R. Sellakumar, and S. A. Borg, *Cancer,* **20**, 857 (1967).

18. W. Bollag, *Eur. J. Cancer,* **8**, 689 (1972).

19. J. E. Smith, P. O. Milch, Y. Muto, and D. S. Goodman, *Biochem. J.,***132**, 821 (1973).

20. J. E. Dowling and G. Wald, *Proc. Natl. Acad. Sci. USA* **46,** 587 (1960).

21. D. S. Goodman, J. E. Smith, R. M. Hembry, and J. T. Dingle. *J. Lipid Res.,* **15**, 406 (1974).

22. W. Bollag, *Eur. J. Cancer.* **10**, 731 (1974).

23. W. Bollag, *Chemotherapy* (Basel), **21**, 236 (1975).

24. C. D. Port, M. B. Sporn, and D. G. Kaufman, *Proc. Am. Assn. Cancer Res.,* **16**, 21 (1975).

25. C. J. Grubbs, R. C. Moon, M. B. Sporn, and D. L. Newton, *Cancer Res.,* in press.

26. M. B. Sporn, R. A. Squire, C. C. Brown, J. M. Smith, M. L. Wenk, and S. Springer, *Science,* in press.

27. P. Nettesheim and M. L. Williams, *Int. J. Cancer,* **17**, 351 (1976).

28. S. M. Cohen, J. F. Wittenberg, and G. T. Bryan, *Cancer Res.,* **36**,2334 (1976).

29. R. M. Hicks and J. S. Wakefield, *Chem.-Biol. Interact.,* **5**, 139 (1972).

30. D. Schmahl, C. Kruger, and P. Preissler, *Arzneim. Forsch.,* **22**,946 (1972).

31. R. C. Moon, C. J. Grubbs, and M. B. Sporn, *Cancer Res.,* **36**, 2626 (1976).

32. S. B. Wolbach and C. L. Maddock, *Proc. Soc. Exp. Biol. Med.,* **77**,825 (1951).

33. M. B. Sporn, N. M. Dunlop, D. L. Newton, and W. R. Henderson, *Nature,* **263**, 110 (1976).

34. J. N. Thompson and G. A. J. Pitt, *Biochim. Biophys. Acta,* **78**,753 (1963).

35. S. Narindrasorasak, P. Pimpa, and M. R. Lakshmanan, *Biochem. J.,* **122**,427 (1971).

10

Taste and Feeding Behavior in Patients with Cancer

WILLIAM D. DEWYS, M.D.

Northwestern University Medical School Chicago, Ill.

Anorexia (reduced appetite or decreased caloric intake or both) is an important determinant of cancer cachexia (1). The pathophysiology of anorexia is not clearly understood but recent observations (2,3) suggest that changes in taste sensation in patients with malignancy may be an important determinant of anorexia. These changes include an elevated threshold for sweet taste and a lowered threshold for bitter taste. In a small series of patients we have correlated decreased caloric intake with these alterations in taste sensation (4). Our data on taste sensation plus patient comments lead to suggestions for modifying the patients' diet which may result in improved caloric intake.

PATIENTS AND METHODS

A series of 50 patients with a spectrum of malignancies of variable extent was studied (2,3). A patient's symptoms were evaluated with a semistructured interview and taste sensation was measured using the technique of Henkin (5,6). Control values for detection and recognition threshold on taste testing were obtained from 17 normal volunteers and six patients with nonneoplastic diseases. In 40 patients of the original series of 50 we estimated daily caloric intake based on a five-day log of food intake with conversion of this food intake information to caloric values by reference

Supported in part by contract #NO1 CP 65779 from the National Cancer Institute.

to standard tables of food composition (7). Data were subjected to signifiance testing using the rank sum test or Chi square with Yates correction (8).

RESULTS

Subjective symptoms elicited on interview included a general reduction in the pleasurable aspect of taste noted by 25 patients with descriptions such as "food tastes blah" and "food has no taste." A majority of these patients equated reduced taste sensation with reduced appetite. Sixteen patients reported an aversion for meat and this group included 13 patients who had also indicated a general reduction in taste sensation and three patients who reported only an aversion for meat.

Evaluation of results from taste testing showed detection and recognition thresholds for NaCl and HCl which were essentially similar in the control and tumor patient group, and these will not be discussed further (2,3). The detection threshold for sucrose showed an upward skewing in the tumor patient group compared to the control population and this difference between patients and controls was also seen for recognition threshold. Seventeen tumor patients had sucrose recognition thresholds above 90 mmole/liter while only one control had a value this high ($\chi^2 = 59.4$ $p < .001$). These abnormalities on sucrose testing for the cancer patients could be correlated with the symptom of decreased taste sensation. Cancer patients who did not have this symptom had sucrose recognition results quite comparable to the controls, with a similar median (60 mmole/liter) and a nearly similar range. In the patients with the symptom of decreased taste sensation, 12 of 25 had recognition thresholds above 90 mmole/liter compared with five of 25 above 90 mmole/liter in the asymptomatic patient group ($\chi^2 = 3.2, p < .08$) and one of 23 in the control group ($\chi^2 = 7.8, p < .01$). Looked at another way, the data show that ten tumor patients had a sucrose recognition threshold above 150 mmole/liter and nine of these reported the symptom of a loss of taste for food ($\chi^2 = 6.1, p < .02$).

The results of testing with urea demonstrated a downward skewing in the tumor patients, with eight tumor patients having recognition thresholds below 90 mmole/liter compared with only one control who had a value this low ($\chi^2 = 10.5, p < .005$). The urea testing results for the cancer patients were divided as to the presence or absence of the symptom of aversion for meat. The majority of patients with this symptom had low urea thresholds, with a median of 75 mmole/liter compared to the median of 300 mmole/liter in the controls and 600 mmole/liter in the patients not having this symptom. In the patients who reported meat aversion, 12 out of 16 had urea recognition thresholds below 300 mmole/liter, which was significantly different from the two out of 34 in the patients denying this symptom ($\chi^2 = 22.5, p < .001$) or the four out of 23 in the control group ($\chi^2 = 10.7, p < .002$).

The relationship between the symptoms of loss of taste or meat aversion and the recognition thresholds for urea and sucrose have been analyzed (3). It was possible to identify four subgroups of patients for the presence or absence of these two symptoms and to correlate the symptom grouping with taste testing results. A group of three patients reported only an aversion for meat, and their taste test results disclosed a low urea threshold and a normal sucrose threshold. Both symptoms were reported by 13 patients and their taste test results revealed a low urea and a high sucrose threshold with some overlap of the normal range. A group of 12 patients reported only a general loss of taste and these patients had a sucrose threshold that was above the normal range (six patients) or above the normal median (the other six), while the urea threshold was normal or elevated. The group denying these two symptoms (22 patients) had thresholds for urea and sucrose which were, with one exception, within the normal range.

The probability of having an abnormality of taste could be correlated with the extent of tumor involvement (3). A group of nine patients with limited disease had normal recognition thresholds for both sucrose and urea. An intermediate group of 21 patients had slightly more advanced disease and three of these had an abnormality of recognition for either sucrose or urea. Patients with advanced disease had a very high probability of having an abnormality of taste sensation, with 15 out of 20 having an abnormality of recognition for sucrose or urea or both (see Table I). This correlation of taste abnormality with advanced disease is highly significant ($p < .001$).

In 40 patients of this series of 50 we obtained data on daily caloric intake. To allow for differences in body size, caloric intake was expressed as calories per kilogram body weight per day (see Fig. 1). Patients whose taste test results were within normal range were subdivided into two groups as to the presence or absence of other factors that might decrease caloric intake. Patients with symptoms of pain, nausea, bowel obstruction, or brain metastases had significant reduction in caloric intake compared with patients not having these symptoms (column 2 vs. column 1 in Fig. 1; $p < .02$). Patients with an abnormally low urea threshold had caloric intakes that were significantly lower than the asymptomatic normal taste group (column 3 vs. column 1; $p < .02$) and also lower than the total group with normal taste (compare column 3

Table 1 Correlation between Tumor Extent and Incidence of Taste Abnormality

Tumor Extent[a]	Normal Taste Threshold	Abnormal Taste Threshold
Limited	9	0
Moderate	18	3
Extensive	5	15

[a]Tumor extent was scored on a 0 to 3 scale by organ site and the sum of all organ scores was called the tumor extent score. Patients with limited extent had scores of 1-2, moderate 3-4, and extensive 5 or more.

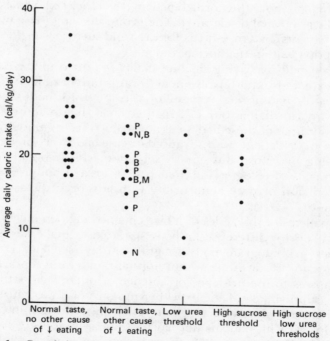

Figure 1. Correlation of caloric intake and taste test results in cancer patients.

with column 1 + 2; $p < .03$). In the group with an elevated sucrose threshold several patients had low caloric intake but this distribution did not reach statistical signifiance compared to the asymptomatic patient group. One patient who had an abnormal low urea threshold and an abnormally high sucrose threshold had a normal caloric intake. This patient was noteworthy in being highly motivated and was apparently able to maintain caloric intake in spite of altered taste sensation. When all the patients with altered taste sensation are lumped together their caloric intake was significantly lower than the asymptomatic group (column 3, 4, 5 vs. column 1; $p < .02$). The comparison between all patients with abnormal taste sensation and all patients with normal taste sensation approached statistical significance (column 1 + 2 vs. columns 3, 4, 5; $p = .07$).

DISCUSSION

The present studies suggest that abnormalities of taste sensation may be an important physiological determinant of the anorexia of malignancy. The hedonic value of taste influences normal food intake behavior and decreased or altered hedonic input may result in decreased caloric intake in the cancer patient. In addition to hedonic considerations one must consider the physiologic effects of taste stimuli. A positive taste stimulus triggers multiple physiologic reflexes, many of which are contributory to the intake and digestion of food. Positive taste stimuli such as sweet stimuli result in the flow of saliva and an increase in gastric secretions (9,10). Positive orogastric stimuli also cause a variety of physiological changes conducive to food intake, including alterations in respiratory quotient and blood glucose (11).

Sweet taste is positive stimulus for the above physiologic reflexes and elevation of the threshold for sweet taste may result in decreased triggering of the reflexes. The taste of acid or bitter normally causes blunting of the above-mentioned physiologic reflexes and a lowering of the taste threshold for bitter may result in more strongly inhibitory effects on these physiologic reflexes.

In management of the anorectic cancer patient one must consider tumor reductive therapy and symptomatic therapy as two possible approaches. Since the likelihood of a taste abnormality correlates with the extent of the tumor, one would expect that response to antineoplastic treatment might result in reduction of these taste abnormalities. Preliminary data support this conclusion. In nine patients in whom a taste abnormality was observed before therapy, and who subsequently responded to therapy with reduction in their tumor burden, there was a trend toward normalization of taste abnormalities. Four patients showed change from a low urea threshold toward normal values and five patients changed from high normal or elevated value for sucrose toward normal values (2).

In considering symptom-directed therapy in patients with an elevated sucrose recognition threshold we have recommended increased sweetening or increased seasoning of food and in a few patients we have been impressed with improvements in caloric intake following this suggestion. Patients with meat aversion often note gradations in this symptom related to the type of meat offered. Calling this to the patient's attention may result in improved protein intake. Patients appear to have greater difficulty in eating beef or pork and less difficulty with poultry or fish. Patients with a more severe abnormality may also have difficulty in eating poultry or fish, but intake of eggs or mild cheeses may still be possible and this change in food selection may permit better protein intake.

Future studies should delineate the time course of development of these taste abnormalities and the time course of the effect of altered taste sensation on caloric intake. Future investigations should also attempt to delineate other factors such as personality and motivational factors which may determine why some patients with abnormal taste sensation have reduced caloric intake while others do not. And finally research to elucidate the pathophysiology of these alterations may permit the development of specific intervention strategies.

REFERENCES

1. C. Waterhouse, *J.Chron.Dis.*, **16**, 6637 (1963).

2. W. D. DeWys, *Ann.N.Y.Acad.Sci.* **230**:427 (1974).

3. W. D. DeWys and K. Walters, *Cancer* **36**, 1888 (1975).

4. W. D. DeWys, "Changes in Taste Sensation in Cancer Patients: Correlation with Caloric Intake," in M. Kare, Ed., *Proceedings of the Second International Conference on the Chemical Senses and Nutrition 1976,* in press.

5. R. I. Henkin, J. R. Gill, F. C. Barter, *J.Clin.Invest.* **42**, 727(1963).

6. R. I. Henkin, P. J. Schechter, R. Hoye, and C. F. T. Mattern, *J.A.M.A.* **217**,434 (1971).

7. *Composition of foods.* Agriculture Handbook #8 USDA, Dec. 1963.

8. A. B. Hill, *Principles of Medical Statistics,* Oxford University Press, New York (1961) p. 172.

9. M. R. Kare, "Digestive Functions of Taste Stimuli," in C. Pfaffmann, Ed., *Olfaction and Taste.* Rockefeller University Press, New York (1969), pp. 586–592.

10. I. P. Pavlov, *The Work of the Digestive Glands,* 2nd ed., Charles Griffin & Co., Ltd., London (1910).

11. S. Nicholaidis, *Ann.N.Y.Acad.Sci.* **157**, 1176 (1969).

11

Effect of Nutrition as Related to Radiation and Chemotherapy

SARAH S. DONALDSON, M.D.

Stanford University School of Medicine, Stanford, California

The importance of diet and nutrition as related to cancer has been recognized since physicians first recorded observations regarding patients. As long ago as the 5th century B.C., Hippocrates wrote

> ... for extreme diseases ... extreme methods of cure, are most suitable ... . when a person is recovering from a disease, has a good appetite, but his body weight does not improve in condition, it is a bad symptom .... we must consider, in which cases food is to be given once or twice a day, and in greater or smaller quantities, and at intervals (1).

This historical writing is applicable to the nutritional concerns associated with aggressive radiation therapy and chemotherapy of the 20th century.

In observations on 500 cancer patients, Dr. Shields Warren noted that greater than 22% of patients died from no other identifiable cause than cachexia of cancer (2). Cancer cachexia and resultant malnutrition are characterized by a triad of systemic manifestations:

1. anorexia with diminished food intake,
2. hypermetabolism for the nutritional state of the individual,
3. wasting of body tissues (3).

Supported in part by Public Health Service Research Grant CA-05838, from the National Cancer Institute, National Institutes of Health, Bethesda, Maryland.

These factors may be compounded by mechanical problems of the gastrointestinal tract which cause decreased absorption, or by infection which increases the energy needs of the host. The tumor itself may trap nutrients at the expense of the host, providing a "nitrogen trap" (4). Thus, the neoplasm ultimately has a unique effect on its host. The oncologist is therefore faced initially with nutritional problems resulting from the tumor, which soon may be intensified by additional nutritional alterations resulting from radiation therapy and chemotherapy used to treat the tumor. The purpose of this chapter is to review dietary and nutritional problems related to radiation therapy and chemotherapy, and to provide therapeutic approaches to help manage these problems.

RADIATION THERAPY

Radiation therapy delivered to any portion of the gastrointestinal tract may create nutritional disorders, either directly or indirectly, by its effect on associated normal tissues as well as on the neoplasm. Eighty-eight to 92% of patients undergoing high-dose radiation to the head and neck and abdominal-pelvic areas experience significant weight loss during treatment when no specific dietary therapy is provided (5). Eight to 13% of such patients suffer a loss of greater than 10% of their body weight between the initiation and the completion of radiotherapy, an approximate six to eight week course of treatment. Many patients are malnourished even prior to the initiation of therapy, which further magnifies the degree of malnutrition.

Nutritional problems are related to the region being irradiated, for example, the head and neck area, the mediastinum, when the esophagus is included within the primary path of the X-ray beam, the abdomen, and the pelvis. Table 1 lists some of the more common problems resulting from radiation therapy which may contribute to nutritional difficulties. Mucositis, stomatitis, gingivitis, and esophagitis resulting from radiation to the upper gastrointestinal tract lead to a decreased oral intake. Radiation alterations on the taste sensors affect feeding behavior and have a great impact on a patient's appetite and eating. Xerostomia resulting from radiation effect on the major and minor salivary glands intensifies difficulties in eating and contributes to dental decay, further complicating eating habits. Dysphagia, anorexia, nausea, and vomiting result in decreased food intake. Radiation enteritis may lead to malabsorption, obstruction, fistula, stricture, ulceration, or perforation and thus affect the patient's nutritional balance (6,7).

The incidence of severe bowel complications secondary to high-dose

Table 1   Sequelae of Radiotherapy Leading to Nutritional Problems

During Treatment	Posttreatment
Anorexia	
Loss of taste	Altered taste
Xerostomia	Xerostomia
	Poor dentition
Mucositis	Mandibular necrosis
Dysphagia	
Nausea and vomiting	Ulcer
Diarrhea	
Acute enteritis	Chronic enteritis

abdominal-pelvic radiation therapy ranges between 11 and 24% in large consecutive series of patients (8,9). Radiation to the gastrointestinal tract continually affects epithelial lining cells, causing a denudation of these rapidly dividing cells. In the small bowel this appears as an alteration of the lining cells of Crypts of Lieberkuhn, leading to a shortening of the crypts, loss of architecture, with ultimate complete distortion and loss of absorptive surface and villi. Although initial exposure may be rapidly repaired (10), repeated exposure to high-dose radiation ultimately causes a submucosal fibrosis with bizarre fibroblast formation which is responsible for scarring. In addition one may see vascular changes among arterioles and arteries with intimal thickening and thrombosis, contributing to ulcer formation and inflammation. Such severe bowel damage may ultimately necessitate surgical resection for alleviation of symptoms.

CHEMOTHERAPY

Nearly all chemotherapeutic agents adversely affect dietary intake. Table 2 summarizes some of the commonly used drugs and their direct or indirect nutritional sequelae. Anorexia is commonly seen as is mucosal ulceration, presenting as mucositis, cheilosis, glossitis, stomatitis, and esophagitis. Virtually all drugs cause nausea and vomiting; many cause diarrhea. Constipation may occur. Some drugs, such as nitrogen mustard and cyclophosphamide, cause an abnormal or metallic taste in the mouth. Vincristine may cause jaw pain; corticosteroid hormones may contribute to ulcer formation.

Table 2   Chemotherapeutic Agents Affecting Dietary Intake

Drugs	Ano-rexia	Mucosal Ulcer-ation	Nausea	Vomit-ing	Diar-rhea	Other
Actinomycin D	+	+	+	+	+	Hepatic dysfunction
Bleomycin	+	+	+	+		
Cyclophosphamide	+		+	+		Altered taste
Cytarabine	+	+	+	+	+	
Doxorubicin		+	+	+	+	
5-fluorouracil	+	+	+	+	+	
Hydroxyurea	+	+	+	+	+	Constipation
Melphalan			+	+		
6-mercaptopurine	+	+	+	+		Hepatic dys-function
Methotrexate	+	+	+	+	+	Hepatic dys-function
Nitrogen mustard	+		+	+	+	Metallic taste
Nitrosoureas	+		+	+		
Vinblastine	+	+	+	+	+	Constipation
Vincristine			+	+		Constipation

The deleterious effect of each of these single agents on the patient's nutritional balance may be accentuated in combination chemotherapy programs. The addition of chemotherapy to radiotherapy increases normal tissue injury. This has been documented in the head and neck (11), esophagus (12,13), and abdomen and pelvic regions (14). Phillips and Fu have summarized the normal tissue injury seen with many of the commonly employed chemotherapeutic agents when combined with radiation therapy (15). The antibiotic chemotherapeutic agents actinomycin D, adriamycin, and bleomycin are most likely to enhance radiation injury. These effects may be particularly severe in the gastrointestinal tract, a rapid cell renewal system that exhibits significant augmentation of radiation injury by a range of cancer chemotherapeutic agents including actinomycin D, adriamycin, and 5-fluorouracil.

Recall of radiation effects has been described with both actinomycin D (11) and adriamycin (16) when given following radiation therapy. Thus, the potential exists for reactivated nutritional problems with each cycle of chemotherapy. Clinicians must take into account such enhanced tissue injury with its expected nutritional sequelae when planning multimodal therapy.

ORAL, DENTAL, AND SYSTEMIC THERAPEUTIC MEASURES

The therapeutic modalities available to treat nutritional problems accompanying radiation or chemotherapy conventionally are administered during the treatment as symptomatic general supportive therapy. They may also be administered prior to treatment, to prepare the patient for radiation or drug treatment or may be given following treatment, to reverse the symptoms created by the treatment. Commonly employed oral and dental therapy is shown in Table 3. Attention to dental care is of utmost importance in a patient receiving radiotherapy to the head and neck region, or to one receiving drug treatment which may cause irritation to the oral mucosa. Such dental attention demands a dental evaluation prior to treatment, with consideration for dental repair or extraction if teeth are carious, compulsive dental hygiene such as teeth and gum brushing, use of dental floss, and fluoride treatment. Mouth washes and oral lavage using gravity drainage or a water pik or both are important. Dilute hydrogen peroxide solutions or salt and soda solutions are most effective in keeping the mouth free of thickened oral secretions which serve as a nidus for bacterial attack if not removed. Local analgestic solutions given as mouth washes or gargles are frequently helpful before meal time if a patient experiences dysphagia. Salivary stimulants with sugarless gum or lemon drops or salivary substitutes may be of use when radiation to the salivary glands changes normal

Table 3   Oral and Dental Therapy

Fluid and electrolytes

Oral hygiene measures
    Mouthwashes and oral irrigations
        H_2O_2 solution
        Salt and soda
    Use of gravity drainage and/or water pik

Salivary substitutes

Dental evaluation
    Repair or extraction
    Teeth and gum cleaning
    Fluoride treatments
    Dental floss
    Trismus exercises

Avoidance of alcohol and tobacco

salivary flow. It is important to avoid any irritants such as alcohol or tobacco, or excessively hot foods.

Various medications, listed in Table 4, may be of use in minimizing acute reactions and in preventing complications. Prompt antibiotic therapy should be used following appropriate cultures when a patient becomes febrile while neutropenic from systemic chemotherapy. Antibiotic use may be of aid to the patient undergoing radiation to the head and neck area, or to the small or large bowel, particularly if there is a history of associated inflammatory bowel disease. Either local or systemic analgesics may be helpful. Liberal use of available compounds providing antiemetic, antispasmodic, anticholinergic, and antidiarrheal action should be provided. Corticosteroid therapy may be of help locally or systemically for reversal of acute and occasionally chronic tissue injury.

DIETARY SUPPORT

Dietary therapy may be utilized in nutritionally depleted cancer patients undergoing aggressive radiation therapy or chemotherapy or both. Table 5 lists dietary therapies that are used. The conventional approach

Table 4   Medications

Antibiotics
Analgesics, local and systemic
Anabolics
Antiemetics
Antispasmodics/anticholinergics
Antidiarrheals
Corticosteroids
Tranquilizers
Vitamins

Table 5   Dietary Modalities

Diets
Soft
Low-residue
Liquid
Diet supplements
Tube feeding
Defined formula diet
Total parenteral nutrition — hyperalimentation

has been to prescribe foods a patient can tolerate. Such dietary therapy may be dictated by previous surgical procedures necessitating a certain consistency of foodstuffs, or a particular route of administration. For example, a liquid or soft diet may be necessary because of the patient's impaired ability to swallow solids. Various dietary supplements are used in an attempt to increase caloric intake. If the patient cannot swallow, tube feedings must be considered. Tube feedings may be given by a nasogastric tube, esophagostomy tube, gastrostomy tube, or a jejunostomy tube depending on the individual clinical situation.

A diet free of gluten, free of milk and milk products, low in fat, and low in residue, given by a slow, continuous drip or in fractionated feedings was used in children with partial to complete small bowel obstruction from radiation and chemotherapy damage to the small bowel (14). The children with chronic radiation enteritis reported in this study all responded dramatically commensurate with receiving specific dietary therapy *alone*, and all have proven to be long-term survivors, suffering no relapses of disease, or recurrent bouts of intermittent intestinal obstruction. This dietary therapy was initiated when the children became malnourished on normal diets and when surgical exploration demonstrated bowel obstruction due to fibrosis, but no evidence of tumor. In each case small bowel radiographs confirmed a radiographic picture of bowel damage including dilated and constricted loops of small bowel, with thickened mucosal folds, and separation of the bowel loops. Jejunal biopsies, prior to dietary therapy, revealed a histologic picture similar to that seen in malabsorption, with subtotal villous atrophy, dilatation of lymphatic vessels, and a moderately dense inflammatory infiltrate in the lamina propria. The specific dietary therapy was gradually supplemented to a normal diet, as tolerated, when radiographs and follow-up small bowel biopsies confirmed repair of the acute mucosal and submucosal changes. The rationale for this therapy was to limit gluten, milk, and milk products when the histologic picture revealed complete villous atrophy and a loss of absorptive surface of the bowel. Fat was limited because of the observed lymphatic dilatation; residue was limited to prevent further mechanical obstruction. The children studied *all* responded dramatically to the dietary treatment alone with relief of bowel obstruction. The dramatic therapeutic effectiveness of this specific diet has now prompted its use as prophylactic therapy in children considered at high risk of bowel damage when abdominal radiation and chemotherapy are administered simultaneously. Since the initiation of the preventive use of this dietary therapy, there have been no cases of severe acute enteritis or delayed enteritis at the Institut Gustave-Roussy (personal communication, J. Lemerle and O. Schweisguth), whereas prior to its use, the incidence was 70% and 36%, respectively.

DEFINED FORMULA DIET

Recently interest has been directed to the use of enteral feeding of defined formula diets. The name "elemental diet" came into use to describe diets in which protein is present in a predigested or elemental form (protein hydrolysate or synthetic amino acids), and carbohydrate and limited fat are present in readily digested forms. Such defined formula diets are almost totally absorbed in the upper gastrointestinal tract and are relatively bulk-free. These diets do not stimulate digestive juices, and being formulated as low in residue, cut down on stool and decrease the number and type of fecal bacteria. A large number of commercially prepared liquid formulas are now on the market, varying greatly in composition and cost. These products have been summarized according to nutritional content, fiber, lactose, amino acid sources, and other nutrients (17). A number of reports in the surgical literature document the use of these diets in the treatment of patients with fistulas of the alimentary tract (18–24), inflammatory bowel disease (20–25), short bowel syndrome (20, 22–24), pancreatitis (20, 21, 23, 26), and various other surgical conditions in critically ill patients (21–24). Enteral feeding has been shown to produce a positive nitrogen balance, weight gain, and restoration of lean body tissue and fat in nutritionally depleted patients, and compares favorably with intravenous feeding (27). Table 6 summarizes some examples of reports of enteral feeding in patients with a variety of intestinal conditions. Weight gain and rise in total protein levels are documented in patients given defined formula dietary therapy as the main or sole nutritional source for prolonged periods.

Because of documented benefit in surgical patients in severe catabolic states, defined formula feeding was extended to nutritionally depleted cancer patients. Much of the experience among patients with neoplastic disease has been gained by Bounous and co-workers, who have treated patients being given defined formula dietary therapy while undergoing radiation therapy and chemotherapy (28, 29). They have demonstrated protection against radiation enteropathy by use of a defined formula diet given throughout the course of radiation therapy (28). Their results are shown in Table 7. Study patients given an elemental diet gained weight and maintained serum protein levels, while control patients given normal diets lost weight and had a decrease in serum protein levels. In addition, control patients experienced more symptomatic diarrhea, three of nine patients requiring an interruption of radiation for 10 to 12 days because of these symptoms. These authors speculated that possible mechanisms of radioprotection included a reduction of pancreatic enzymes and secretions by a substitution of proteins by amino acids, and

Table 6   Elemental Dietary Therapy

Reference	Number of Patients	Indication	Diet	Duration	Change in Body Weight	Change in Total Protein
(24)	11	Preoperative preparation Fistula Short bowel syndrome Obstruction	Vivonex HN (Eaton)	3-16 weeks	+10.6 lbs	+0.5
(22)	9	Regional enteritis	Flexical (Mead-Johnson)	8-27 days (av. 16 d)	+ 1.8 lbs.	
(19)	13	Alimentary tract fistulas	Codelid and Vivonex	5-50 days	+ 7.7 lbs.	+0.5

Table 7 Dietary Therapy during Radiotherapy [a]

	Number of Patients	Radiation Dose/ Time in Days	Changes in Body Weight	Symptoms	Mean Serum Protein
Controls					
Normal diets	9	2000R/15D to 5040R/42D	− 3.5 lbs.	6/9 diarrhea (3 severe)	↓
Study Patients					
Elemental diet Flexical (Mead-Johnson)	9	3000R/22D to 5800R/40D	+ 1.6 lbs.	1/9 diarrhea	No change

[a] Data from (28).

more efficient absorption of these amino acids by the irradiated bowel. They also noted the importance of median chain triglycerides, which have been shown to enhance fat absorption in humans with radiation bowel damage (30). These authors concluded that nutritional status and perhaps the immunologic status of cancer patients could be maintained *during* intensive irradiation by use of a carefully administered defined formula diet. The next obvious question to be answered is whether it is possible to protect against late radiation damage by prophylactic administration of a defined formula diet to patients undergoing intensive radiation to the small bowel. A clinical trial is currently underway at Stanford University Medical Center to investigate this possibility.

Bounous and co-workers have extended their investigations to study the effect of an elemental diet in patients undergoing chemotherapy, specifically patients with metastatic carcinoma receiving 5-fluorouracil (5-FU) (29). The use of 5-FU has been demonstrated to produce specific histologic abnormalities of the colonic and rectal mucosa (31, 32). Bounous and investigators studied the clinical and histologic findings during 5-FU therapy among patients receiving normal hospital diets, compared to comparable patients receiving an elemental diet. Table 8 summarizes the findings in this study. No difference in total caloric intake was demonstrated between the two groups; however, there was a higher caloric intake in the treated group when expressed per kilogram of body weight. No weight loss occured among the treated group. They noted a striking difference in the surface epithelium of the rectum, with the preservation of the epithelial cells in those patients receiving dietary therapy, and postulated that the substitution of amino acids for whole protein in the chemically defined diet is responsible for this protection as a result of increased intestinal absorption of the amino acids.

Studies using other chemotherapeutic agents known to have gastrointestinal toxicity, such as adriamycin, actinomycin D, high dose velban, and methotrexate will be important to further investigate a possible beneficial role of defined formula dietary therapy during intensive cytotoxic drug treatment.

Complications of defined formula dietary therapy include hyperglycemia, hyperosmolar dehydration, and hypertonic nonketotic coma. Administration of the hypertonic solution may create gastric retention, and nausea and diarrhea may occur. Careful attention to fluid and electrolyte balance is essential during treatment. These diets, low in fat, are often found to be unpalatable, and attention to flavorings and mixture with various juices to camouflage the taste are important. They are best served cold, as a drink or slush, sipped slowly to prevent cramping, flatulence, and diarrhea from the hyperosmolar load. The diet should

Table 8 Dietary Therapy during Chemotherapy 5-FU [a]

	Number of Patients	Total Dose 5-FU (gm)	Duration of 5-FU	Mean cal/Day during 5-FU	Mean Body Weight	Mean cal/kg Body Weight	Mean Height of Surface Epithelium of Rectum after 5-FU (μ)
Controls Normal hospital food	12	3.82	6-9 days	1639	− 2.77 Kg.	20.4 Kcal/Kg	42.1
Study Patients Elemental diet Flexical (Mead-Johnson)	9	4.01	6-9 days	1725	No change	27.1 Kcal/Kg	58.1

[a] Data from (29).

initially be diluted to one-half strength or less, gradually increased to three-fourths strength, and ultimately to full strength, to prevent symptoms from the hyperosmolar load. Sufficient fluids should be given to maintain an adequate urinary output and provide electrolyte balance.

TOTAL PARENTERAL NUTRITION

During the past decade the techniques of intravenous feeding have been developed to make possible continuous long-term delivery of protein hydrolysates and hypertonic glucose into the superior vena cava by a catheter. Thus the administration of concentrated nutrient solutions not tolerated by peripheral veins is possible. The word parenteral means access to the body other than by the enteral or intestinal tract. This technique of intravenous hyperalimentation can provide nutrients in quantities beyond basal requirements and thus achieve positive nitrogen balance.

The initial experience with intravenous hyperalimentation (IVH) came in surgical patients with nutritional requirements far in excess of what could be administered with conventional intravenous therapy. These included patients undergoing major operative procedures, those with burns or with major trauma, and those with intestinal obstruction, gastrointestinal fistulae, and inflammatory lesions of the bowel (33–37). It was soon demonstrated that with careful attention to proper catheter placement, complications could be minimized and patients could be maintained safely for prolonged periods (27). A strict protocol for aseptic technique of catheter placement and maintenance of the catheter by a specially trained team lowers the rate of contamination and sepsis. In large studies the risk of catheter-related contamination was only 7.3%, and catheter-related clinical sepsis only 2.2% (38,39). In careful hands IVH has been shown to be safe even in cancer patients with neutropenia and impaired resistance to infection (40). Most complications of IVH are technical and include those related to placement of the central venous catheter, such as pneumothorax, hydrothorax, hemothorax, hydromediastinum, central venous thrombophlebitis, air embolism, catheter embolism, catheter misplacement, injury to the subclavian artery, thoracic duct, or bracheal plexus. The third area of concern is metabolic complications related to the improper formulation or administration of the fluid, hyperosmolar dehydration, hyperglycemia, hypoglycemia, hypercalcemia, hypophosphatemia, hyperchloremic metabolic acidosis, hyponatremia, or hypernatremia. When proper attention is paid to the patient's metabolic state, these complications are rare (41).

During the past five years, much experience has been gained in parenteral hyperalimentation of cancer patients. It has most often been used for presurgical and postsurgical therapy, and for metabolic support of the debilitated patient following surgery, radiation, or chemotherapy. However, the exact role of IVH in patients with malignancy is not yet defined. Some observers report that although patients free of cancer or those with minimal residual disease usually respond well to hyperalimentation, those with extensive cancer are unable to utilize the hyperalimentation solution and experience progressive deterioration (42, 43). Yet others report subjective and objective improvement even among debilitated cancer patients, with an improved performance status, gain in lean body mass, fat deposition, and weight gain commensurate with the parenteral hyperalimentation (44,45).

RESPONSE TO TREATMENT

Total parenteral nutrition has also been shown to be of use in minimizing symptoms related to high-dose radiation therapy and chemotherapy, thus enabling patients to complete a planned course of anticancer therapy without interruption due to poor tolerance of aggressive treatment (46–48).

In addition to apparent increased tolerance to treatment it is possible that added nutritional support may affect response to treatment. Lanzotti and co-workers demonstrated an increased response rate to chemotherapy among debilitated patients with bronchogenic carcinoma treated simultaneously with IVH. In combination chemotherapy with bleomycin, cyclophosphamide, vincristine, methotrexate, and 5-fluorouracil, chemotherapy response (50% reduction in the product of two perpendicular diameters of all measurable lesions) was five of 10 among the high weight loss group of patients treated with IVH as compared to 0 of 12 responses among a historical matched group of patients not treated with IVH (49). Bone marrow toxicity and doses of drug delivered were similar among the two groups. Others have reported the impression of "greater than usual therapeutic responses" to chemotherapy when total parenteral nutrition is used as an adjunct to chemotherapy (50), and support the use of total parenteral nutrition to provide a possible tumor response in patients who otherwise would be denied adequate oncologic therapy because of their cachectic state (51).

Investigators have questioned whether forced feeding might result in increased tumor growth and thus have a deleterious effect on patient survival. Terepka and Waterhouse force-fed patients with widespread malignancy and observed apparent increased tumor growth in some patients during the feeding period (52). Laboratory studies in rodents have also shown the tumor growth occurs more readily in well-nourished than in malnourished animals. For instance, studies on transplanted mammary tumors in rats demonstrated increased rate of tumor growth in rats fed intravenous amino acids and glucose solutions as opposed to rats given only 5% glucose (53). The amino acid treated rats showed better preservation of body mass. It is possible that cell cycle-specific chemotherapeutic agents might be more effective if nutritional support induces an increase in the growth fraction of tumors (51, 53).

SUMMARY

Present cancer treatment modalities, radiotherapy and chemotherapy, cannot be confined exclusively to malignant cell populations. Morbidity to normal tissues, ultimately affecting the nutritional status, must be considered when such therapy is prescribed. It is essential to weigh the potential benefit of treatment against the complications resulting from such therapy. If the nutritional sequelae from such therapy may be effectively treated by attention to nutritional support before, during, and following radiotherapy and chemotherapy, such aggressive forms of therapy may be further justified.

Important questions such as the effect of nutritional support on the neoplasm, the degree of improved tolerance of the patient to anticancer therapy, and protection against normal tissue damage due to anticancer therapy, can only be answered by well-constructed, prospective, randomized clinical trials. Whether attention to nutrition can improve survival and relapse-free survival among patients receiving aggressive anticancer therapy with curative intent is unknown. We must carefully evaluate the *direct* effects of nutritional support on the tumor itself, since it is possible that force feeding a malnourished cancer patient without concomittant effective anticancer therapy might result in an accelerated tumor growth. In addition, we must demonstrate that improved nutrition during a course of radiotherapy and chemotherapy results in an increased tolerance to the treatment, and that such a response is not simply temporary but will result in a long-term effect on survival and disease-free survival rates. It is also important to demonstrate that special attention to nutrition can help *prevent* the anticipated morbidity associated with aggressive radiotherapy and chemotherapy.

REFERENCES

1. Hippocrates. Aphorisms, *in* W. H. S. Jones, *Hippocrates with an English Translation*, Volume IV, Putnam, New York, Heineman, London, (1931), pp. 97–221.

2. S. Warren, *Am. J. Med. Sci.* **184**, 610 (1932).

3. C. Waterhouse, *J. Chron. Dis.* **16**, 637 (1963).

4. J. Mayer, *Postgrad. Med.* **50**, 65 (1971).

5. S. S. Donaldson, Nutritional Consequences of Radiotherapy. *Cancer Res.,* in press.

6. N. J. Greenberger, and K. J. Isselbacher, *Am. J. Med.,* **36**, 450 (1964).

7. W. Duncan and J. C. Leonard, *Quart. J. Med.,* **34**, 319 (1965).

8. D. R. Goffinet, M. J. Schneider, E. Glatstein, H. Ludwig, G. R. Ray, R. Dunnick, and M. A. Bagshaw, *Radiology:* **117**, 149 (1975).

9. B. Hintz, Z. Fuks, R. Kempson, J. Eltringham, C. Zaloudek, T. Williamson, and M. A. Bagshaw, *Radiology,* **114**, 695 (1975).

10. J. S. Trier, and T. H. Browning, *J. Clin. Invest.,* **45**, 194 (1966).

11. S. S. Donaldson, J. R. Castro, J. R. Wilbur, and R. H. Jesse, Jr., *Cancer* **31**, 26 (1973).

12. F. A. Greco, H. S. Brereton, H. Kent, H. Zimbler, J. Merrill, and R. E. Johnson, *Ann. Intern. Med.* **85**, 294 (1976).

13. A. Horwich, J. J. Lokich, and W. D. Bloomer, *Lancet* **2**:561 (1975).

14. S. S. Donaldson, S. Jundt, C. Ricour, D. Sarrazin, J. Lemerle, and O. Schweisguth, *Cancer,* **35**, 1167 (1975).

15. T. L. Phillips, and K. K. Fu, *Cancer* **37**, 1186 (1976).

16. S. S. Donaldson, J. M. Glick, and J. R. Wilbur, *Ann. Intern. Med.* **81**, 407(1974).

17. M. E. Shils, A. S. Bloch, and R. Chernoff, *Clin. Bull.,* **6**:151 (1976).

18. A. J. Voitk, V. Echave, R. A. Brown, A. H. McArdle, and F. N. Gurd, *Surg. Gynecol. Obstet.,* **137**, 68 (1973).

19. K. D. Bury, R. V. Stephens, and H. T. Randall, *Am. J. Surg.* **121**, 174 (1971).

20. A. J. Voitk, R. A. Brown, A. H. McArdle, E. J. Hinchey, and F. N. Gurd, *C.M.A. J.,* **107**, 123 (1972).

21. J. Rivard, and R. Lapointe, *Can. J. Surg.,* **18**, 90 (1975).

22. G. Bounous, G. Devroede, H. Haddad, R. Beaudry, B. Perey, and L. Lejeune, *Dis. Col. Rect.,* **17**, 157 (1974).

23. R. V. Stephens, and H. T. Randall, *Ann. Surg.,* **170**, 642 (1969).

24. T. F. Nealon, C. E. Grossi, and M. Streier, *Ann. Surg.,* **180**, 9 (1974).

25. A. J. Voitk, V. Echave, J. H. Feller, R. A. Brown, and F. N. Gurd, *Arch. Surg.,* **197**, 329 (1973).

26. A. Voitk, R. A. Brown, V. Echave, A. H. McArdle, F. N. Gurd, and A. G. Thompson, *Am. J. Surg.* **125**, 223 (1973).

27. D. B. Allardyce, and A. C. Groves, *Surg., Gynecol., Obstet.,* **139**, 179 (1974).

28. G. Bounous, E. Le Bel, J. Shuster, P. Gold, W. T. Tahan, and E. Bastin, *Strahlentherapie,* **149**, 476 (1975).

29. G. Bounous, J. M. Gentile, and J. Hugon, *Can. J. Surg.,* **14**, 312 (1971).

30. H. Haddad, G. Bounous, W. T. Tahan, G. Devroede, R. Beaudry, and R. Lafond, *Dis. Col. Rec.,* **17**, 373 (1974).

31. M. H. Floch, and L. Hellman, *Gastroenterology,* **48**, 430 (1965).

32. S. S. Milles, A. L. Muggia, and H. M. Spiro, *Gastroenterology,* **43**, 391 (1962).

33. S. J. Dudrick, J. M. Long, E. Steiger, and J. E. Rhoads, *Med. Clin. North Am.* **54**, 577 (1970).

34. S. J. Dudrick, and E. M. Copeland, "Parenteral Hyperalimentation" *in* Lloyd M. Myhus, Ed., *Surgery Annual,* Appleton-Century-Crofts, New York (1973), pp. 69–95.

35. B. H. MacPherson, *Am. Surgeon* **35**, 705 (1969).

36. C. W. Van Way, H. C. Meng, and H. H. Sandstead, *Ann. Surg.* **177**, 103 (1973).

37. C. M. Vogel, R. J. Kingsbury, and A. E. Baue, *Arch. Surg.* **105**, 414 (1972).

38. E. M. Copeland, B. V. MacFadyen, C. McGown, and S. J. Dudrick, *Surg., Gynecol., Obstet.,* **138**, 377 (1974).

39. E. M. Copeland, J. M. Daly, and S. J. Dudrick, Nutrition as an adjunct to cancer treatment in the adult. *Cancer Res.,* in press.

40. J. E. Sumners, P. Zee, and W. T. Hughes, *J. Ped.,* **83**, 288 (1973).

41. W. J. Wyrick, W. J. Rea, and R. N. McClelland, *J.A.M.A.* **211**, 1697 (1970).

42. J. H. Ford, R. C. Dudan, J. S. Bennett, and H. E. Averette, *Gynecol. Oncol.* **1**, 70 (1972).

43. R. DeMatteis, and R. E. Hermann, *Cleve. Clin. Quart.* **40**, 139 (1973).

44. E. M. Copeland, B. V. MacFayden, and S. J. Dudrick, *J. Surg. Res.,* **16**, 241 (1974).

45. G. F. Schwartz, H. L. Green, M. L. Bendon, W. P. Graham, and W. S. Blakemore, *Am. J. Surg.,* **121**, 169 (1971).

46. R. M. Filler, N. Jaffe, J. R. Cassady, D. G. Traggis, and J. B. Das, Parenteral nutritional support in children with cancer. *Cancer,* in press.

47. E. M. Copeland, E. A. Suchon, B. V. MacFayden, M. A. Rapp, and S. J. Dudrick, Intravenous hyperalimentation as an adjunct to radiation therapy. *Cancer,* in press.

48. E. M. Copeland, B. V. MacFayden, W. S. MacComb, O. Guillamondegui, R. H. Jesse, and S. J. Dudrick, *Cancer* **35**, 606 (1975).

49. V. J. Lanzotti, E. M. Copeland, S. L. George, S. J. Dudrick, and M. L. Samuels, *Cancer Chemother. Rep.,* **59**, 437 (1975).

50. E. A. Souchon, E. M. Copeland, P. Watson, and S. J. Dudrick, *J. Surg. Res.,* **18**, 451 (1975).

51. E. M. Copeland, B. V. MacFayden, V. J. Lanzotti, and S. J. Dudrick, *Am. J. Surg.,* **129**, 167 (1975).

52. A. R. Terepka and C. Waterhouse, *Am. J. Med.,* **20**, 225 (1956).

53. E. Steiger, J. Oram-Smith, E. Miller, L. Kuo, and H. M. Vars, *J. Surg. Res.* **18**, 455 (1975).

12

Nutrition in the Treatment of Cancer

MAURICE E. SHILS, M.D., Sc.D.

Memorial Sloan-Kettering Cancer Center, Cornell University Medical College, New York, N.Y.

EFFECTS OF SURGICAL INTERVENTION ON NUTRITIONAL STATUS

To meet the needs of the cancer patient adequately, one must know the factors that may adversely affect nutritional status. Such understanding provides the basis for appropriate therapy.

The effects of radiation and of chemotherapy have been reviewed in Chapter 11. In order to complete the review of antitumor treatments, the first portion of this chapter summarizes some of the major effects of surgery. The major procedures and their sequlae that can adversely affect the patient are listed in Table I and discussed briefly below.

Radical surgery of the head and neck to remove cancer has been and continues to be done in frequent conjunction with radiation and now with chemotherapy. Removal of major portions of the tongue, portions of the mouth, mandibles, and chewing muscles often imposes serious functional difficulties in chewing and swallowing. A decrease in salivary secretions leads to dry mouth and adds to the swallowing difficulty, which is exacerbated by radiation with concomitant loss of teeth, pain, and loss of taste and smell (1). These accentuate anorexia, which may further diminish intake. A significant proportion of these patients have an alcoholic history and tend to be malnourished on this basis. The disfiguring surgery is often associated with depression, which further adds to impaired intake. Difficulties in swallowing increase the risk of aspiration of food and secretions with resultant pneumonia. Aspiration can be overcome by laryngectomy but the price of this procedure is loss of voice. Patients with difficulties in swallowing can be taught to improve their ability in this direction by training and by exercise. Such patients

Table 1   Sequelae of Surgery with Adverse Nutritional Effects

1. Resection of oropharyngeal area
   a. Chewing, taste, and swallowing difficulties
   b. Dependency on tube feeding

2. Esophagectomy and restoration of continuity
   a. Vagotomy effects
      - gastric stasis
      - gastric hypochlorhydria
      - diarrhea
      - steatorrhea
   b. Fistula

3. Gastrectomy
   a. Dumping syndrome
   b. Intrinsic factor deficiency
   c. Malabsorption, acute and chronic
   d. Hypoglycemia

4. Intestinal resection
   a. Jejunum
      1. Decreased absorption of many nutrients
   b. Ileum
      1. Vitamin B_{12} deficiency
      2. Conjugated bile salt losses: diarrhea and steatorrhea
      3. Hyperoxaluria; renal oxalate stone
   c. Massive bowel resection
      1. Malabsorption of life-threatening severity
      2. Metabolic acidosis
      3. Gastric hypersecretion
   d. Ileostomy
      1. Complication of salt and water balance
   e. Blind loop syndrome in various situations

5. Pancreatectomy, partial or total
   a. Malabsorption
   b. Diabetes mellitus
   c. Fistula

6. a. Nephrectomy
   b. Cystectomy   —→ renal dysfunction
   c. Ureteral diversion

7. Major hepatic resection
   a. Hypoalbuminemia
   b. Hypoglycemia   —→ postoperative

differ in their ability to manage foods of different textures; many swallow soft foods such as mashed potatoes or thick custards better than thin liquids. Moist foods are more easily swallowed than dry foods.

Many consider the function of the esophagus to be a peristaltic tube from the mouth to the stomach. However, it should be recalled that the vagus nerves are closely associated with the distal esophagus and that distal esophagectomy requires total bilateral vagotomy in cancer patients. Resection of these nerves interrupts neural pathways to the stomach, liver, gallbladder, pancreas, the entire small bowel, and a major portion of the large bowel. Removal of the distal esophagus is done in conjunction with removal of the proximal portion of the stomach. Hypochlorhydria, gastric atony, and a high incidence of diarrhea and steatorrhea occur (2). The hypochlorhydria results in bacterial overgrowth; the gastric atony and small stomach lead to rapid satiety. If a portion of the stomach, small, or large bowel is used to form an artificial esophagus, there is easy reflux since there is no longer the esophagocardiac junction which normally has a sphincter action. These factors are often associated with weight loss. Frequent small meals and liquid formulas and replacement of dietary fat by medium chain triglycerides (MCT) may be helpful.

High subtotal or total gastrectomy causes rapid transit of food into the upper jejunum, and this may lead to the "dumping syndrome." This is manifested in the patient as variable degrees of distressing symptoms, including palpitations, sweating, faintness, and occassional abdominal pains occurring shortly after eating. When the symptoms are severe the patient often becomes fearful of eating, with consequent weight loss (3). Inadequate intake may be complicated by significant steatorrhea consequent to the surgery (4). Removal of intrinsic-factor producing cells leads to the inability to absorb vitamin B_{12}.

The "dumping syndrome" may be markedly decreased or prevented by the ingestion of frequent and small meals of foods with a low osmolality. Injections of vitamin B_{12} prevent deficiency. The rapid entry of food into the small bowel leads to abnormal elevation of serum insulin (5). The rapid absorption and transit of food combined with the loss of the normal reservoir function of the stomach deprives the patient of a sustained source of food. This fact combined with the elevated levels of insulin may lead to hypoglycemic symptoms several hours or more following meal ingestion. This is another reason why the use of frequent meals is desirable in such patients. Deficiencies of calcium, iron, and fat-soluble vitamins may develop with time (6).

Periampullary carcinoma (i.e., in head of pancreas, distal bile duct, duodenum, and ampulla of Vater) is treated by the Whipple procedure, which involves partial gastrectomy, partial (or total) pancreatectomy, duodenectomy, and cholecystectomy and may also involve vagotomy. When partial pancreatectomy is performed and the cut end of the Duct of Wirsung is anastomosed to the jejunum many patients will develop an exocrine pancreatic insufficiency. Ligation of the duct or total pancreatomy obviously results in such pancreatic insufficiency with maldigestion. Diabetes mellitus occurs in a significant proportion of those with partial pancreatectomies. Replacement of digestive enzymes with adequate pancreatic extract will improve the digestion of fats, carbohydrates, and protein. More radical surgery which attempts to remove tumor that has extended beyond the pancreas (so called regional pancreatectomy) leads to further insult to the intestinal tract by removing more small bowel, occasionally large bowel, and by stripping the surface of blood vessels of their accompanying nerves and lymphatic channels (7). The patients have severe nutritional problems (8).

Removal of the jejunum depresses absorption of most nutrients. The hyperplastic compensatory capacity of the remaining ileum is marked provided that postoperative nutritional support is adequate and there is no underlying serious pathology of the vascular system or endothelium. Hence, reasonably good nutritional state can be expected following such compensation if the dietary intake is adequate. Removal of the ileum results in malabsorption of vitamin B_{12} and of conjugated bile salts, since the distal ileum is the physiological site for absorption of these compounds. Lack of absorption of conjugated bile salts results in their entry into the large bowel, where they are deconjugated by bacterial action and where they induce secretion of water and electrolytes into the large bowel with resultant watery diarrhea. The consequences of loss of bile salts and the limited ability of the liver to form new bile salts are a depressed concentration of bile salts in the small bowel with decreased micelle formation and resultant impaired fat absorption (9). When the extent of distal ileal resection is limited, cholestyramine may markedly decrease the diarrhea and a low fat diet or replacement of long chain fats with MCT will decrease the steatorrhea. Vitamin B_{12} deficiency can be avoided by periodic intramuscular injections of this vitamin.

Ileal resection is associated with an increased incidence of hyperoxaluria and renal oxalate calculi, presumably because of increased oxalate absorption (10). Restriction of oxalate-containing foods and oxalate-forming substances is indicated together with close follow-up.

Resection of very large amounts (more than 80%) of both jejunum and ileum is termed massive bowel resection and will result in severe malabsorption in the period postoperatively when the patient begins to eat. The prognosis of the patient will depend on the amount and status of remaining small bowel, the status of the ileocecal valve and colon, the adequacy of the enteric blood supply, and the capacity of the remaining small bowel to develop compensatory hyperplasia. The nutrition management of patients with "short-bowel syndrome" calls for expert and close supervision of the patient (11). It will often require special nutritional therapy beginning with total parenteral nutrition (TPN) and progressing through special tube and oral feedings if sufficient compensation develops. If absorption does not improve to the point where the patient can be sustained on tube or oral feedings, consideration must be given to maintenance or home total parenteral nutrition (12, 13).

Resection of the large bowel, particularly the ascending colon, results in removal of an organ whose primary function is that of water and electrolyte reabsorption and exchange. In most patients there is usually a good degree of adaptation so that the ileostomy drainage is relatively low in water and electrolytes. However, there are some patients who do not adapt and others in whom fluid and electrolyte problems develop during periods of extra fluid loss secondary to enteritis or excessive sweating.

Ureterosigmoidostomy (insertion of ureters into the sigmoid colon) is rarely performed now, having been supplemented by a procedure in which one or both ureters enter a small segment of terminal ileum, one end of which opens on the abdomen (ileal conduit). Ureterosigmoidostomy was abandoned because of the development of hypochloremic metabolic acidosis and hypokalemia. Ileal conduit formation is relatively free of such complications (8).

Major hepatic resection requires adequate nutritional support preoperatively and provision of adequate amounts of albumin and glucose for a limited period in the postoperative period (8).

ENTERAL FEEDING BY TUBE

When oral intake is contraindicated or is inadequate, consideration must be given to the two alternatives—tube feeding or intravenous feeding. Specific contraindications to oral feeding are listed in Table 2.

In situations where the gastrointestinal tract is not functioning (e.g., total intestinal obstruction or persistent vomiting) the only possible alternative is intravenous feeding. In other situations both alternatives are feasible and the final decision must be based on a number of considerations. Some of these considerations are listed in Table 3. They will be reviewed by the physician as he considers the needs of the individual patient. The alternatives are not to be considered in competition with the

Table 2   Contraindications to Oral Feeding

1. Impaired swallowing
2. Obstruction of the alimentary tract
3. Ileus
4. Fistulas, especially of upper alimentary tract
5. Coma
6. Severe malabsorption with massive fluid and electrolyte losses
7. Persistent vomiting

preconceived idea that one is better than the other in all situations where not obviously contraindicated. In general, it is desirable to utilize the alimentary tract if it is functioning adequately. Tube feeding tends to be much less expensive than parenteral feeding and can be conducted much more easily on an outpatient basis as well as an inpatient basis. Entry of food into the alimentary tract is a stimulus to maintenance of structure and function of that tract and to hyperplasia when resection of bowel has occurred.

However, in a situation where a patient has lost the gag reflex, is debilitated, and has significant pulmonary disease, the danger of aspiration during tube feeding is appreciable. In such instances parenteral feeding is desirable.

When a small bowel fistula is such that any kind of oral or tube feeding leads to greater losses of fluid and nutrients through the fistula than are given, then parenteral feeding is obviously preferable. Where a high fistula can be bypassed by the tube or when there is sufficient absorption above or beyond the fistula, feeding by tube may be very efficacious.

Where plans for treatment include cyclical chemotherapeutic agents likely to induce deleterious effects on the mucosa or anorexia or vomit-

Table 3   Alternatives to Oral Feeding: Factors Influencing a Decision

1. Degree and duration of failure in achieving adequate oral intake: The nutritional status of the patient
2. Contraindications to oral intake
3. Safety and potential complications of alternatives
4. Plans for patient treatment
5. Duration of need of alternatives
6. Acceptance of alternatives by patient and family
7. Medical capability in offering alternatives
8. Patient capacity to respond to alternatives
9. Costs to hospital and to patient

ing for protracted periods, parenteral feeding maybe more desirable than the tube feeding. On the other hand, patients with depressed bone marrow, with anorexia, and without vomiting are candidates for tube feeding. For prolonged feeding where there is no contraindication to tube feeding, it is the method of choice.

Either alternative is adequate only if it provides the patient with the necessary calories and nutrients. It has been my experience that all too frequently tube feedings are not given in sufficient amounts even though the proper orders are written. Nurse and house staff will rarely change the rate or volume of infusion of parenteral fluids without good cause but this attitude often does not extend to tube feedings. Attention to this problem by the nutrition team is merited in terms of provision of adequate pumps and education of staff.

Tube Feeding Sites

Figure 1 diagrammatically indicates the four most common positions for tube insertion. Although the *nasopharyngeal tube* is the simplest to insert since it requires no surgical intervention, its use often creates problems. Many cancer patients have had prior experience with nasal tubes and recall too vividly the associated sore throat and difficulty in swallowing during a period of serious illness. It is not surprising that such patients do not wish to have a similar experience. An occasional patient will have a severe depressive reaction upon reinsertion of a tube for feeding purposes. A sympathetic approach and prior agreement to remove the tube if uncomfortable is helpful in overcoming this understandable reservation.

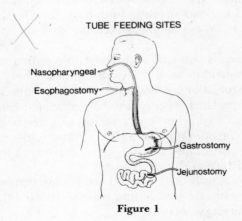

Figure 1

Silicone elastomer (silastic) tubes with small caliber are much better tolerated than the usual rubber or rather firm plastic tube. If the physician can induce the patient to allow the silastic tube to be inserted, the patient will often tolerate the tube for long periods without significant discomfort even in the face of esophagitis. The soft silastic tubes tend to be regurgitated on coughing and may have to be weighted with a small rubber bag containing mercury. A narrow bore tube requires a finely dispersed liquid formulation in order to avoid clogging. The usual home-homogenized tube formula with vegetables, meats, or cereals will not go through such tubes rapidly enough.

The tip of the nasopharyngeal tube is best placed in the lower esophagus so it does not interfere with the normal closure of the esophagogastric junction, which tends to prevent reflux of gastric juice into the esophagus. Rapid feeding through the tube increases the possibility of reflux and the danger of aspiration. Slow feeding over a prolonged period of time using a pump while the patient is in a semisitting position will markedly decrease the possibility of significant reflux. Loss of gag reflex, difficulty in managing secretions, hicupping, significant nausea, and significant pulmonary dysfunction are contraindications to tube feeding.

Placement of an Esophagostomy Tube

This involves surgical insertion of the tube through the neck into the esophagus. The surgery is simple and potentially a much less hazardous procedure than the insertion of a feeding gastrostomy or jejunostomy. It eliminates the psychologic and social problems faced by the outpatient with a nasopharyngeal tube. It is an alternative to a jejunostomy tube for those unobstructed patients needing long-term tube feeding who have subtotal gastrectomy or esophagogastrectomy with the stomach in the chest.

A *feeding gastrostomy* is also a valuable route for feeding through a tube when there is obstruction above the stomach or for long-term feeding when the patient is unwilling to tolerate a nasopharyngeal or esophagostomy tube. When intestinal surgery is to be performed which is likely to result in serious malabsorption, construction of a feeding gastrostomy should be done on the operating table. Simple and reinforced directions to nurses, patient, and family are necessary to prevent leakage and to ensure proper skin care at the entry site.

A *jejunostomy tube* is indicated when there is obstruction more proximally. A final bore catheter for feeding may be inserted through a needle at the time of surgery (14).

Liquid Formulations for Tube Feeding

An important facet of clinical medicine is the liquid formula designed to maintain or improve nutrition by oral or tube administration. In years past, the usual hospital tube feeding formula was based on whole milk, powdered milk, and cream in various combinations. Most noncaucasian adults have insufficient lactase in the intestinal brush border to permit adequate digestion of large amounts of milk. Lactose intolerance occurs also in individuals with gastric or intestinal resection, intestinal radiation damage, and diseases which adversely affect intestinal function. This has led to modifications in the composition of such formulas to ensure adequate nutrition without excessive lactose.

The recent availability of commercial nutritionally complete preparations for oral or tube use is a major step forward. These are derived in whole or in part from natural foods, from food isolates, or from synthetic compounds. These have been given various designations such as "chemically defined"or "elemental" diets. Inasmuch as these diets are usually not "chemically defined" and are not "elemental" in a chemical or physical sense, it has been suggested that they be designated as "defined-formula diets (DFD)" (15). Their development has been stimulated by predictions and claims that such formulations are useful for patients with clinical problems related to the ingestion, digestion, or absorption of solid food.

A large number of commercially prepared formulas are now on the market varying greatly in composition and cost. They differ in completeness, the amounts of "residue" and lactose, and the quantities and sources of amino acids, carbohydrate, and fat. The amino acid sources include intact protein of various types, protein hydrolysate, or free amino acids. Carbohydrates may be polysaccharides, oligosaccharides, disaccharides, or monosaccharides singly or in combination. The fat sources may be long chain polyunsaturated fats or medium chain fats. They vary greatly in palatability for oral use. Details of composition of a large number of such preparations have been published recently (16).

Nutritionally complete defined formula diets are both a boon and a problem to the physician and dietitian. They are easy to store, to order, to prepare, and to administer. However, a serious difficulty may arise from the fact that these formulas are "fixed" in composition. Patients having metabolic problems may be adversely affected by the amounts of one or more nutrients present in the volume necessary to meet overall nutritional requirements. Patients with renal disease may not tolerate the levels of protein, sodium, potassium, phosphate, or magnesium present. Those with hepatic dysfunction may need restrictions in protein and sodium and increased levels of potassium with certain diuretics.

Hyperosmolar nonketotic coma can occur in diabetic patients given inadequate insulin just as well on tube-fed high carbohydrate formulas as with total parenteral nutrition. The dietitian must be aware of the specific composition of formulations available or ordered by a physician and possible contraindications imposed by a clinical situation. The dietitian may modify a formula to meet special needs by either adding desired ingredients or diluting out those that are undesirable and making up the differences in needed constituents from other sources.

Alternatively, formulations to meet the prescription may be made in hospital from individual nutrients. Such individual nutrients are commercially available and can be easily combined to meet the proper medical prescription by a dietitian trained in this field. Manufacturers can also assist in overcoming the limitation of "fixed" formulations by packaging formula diets in "modular"form. In this manner, the most common critical items, such as sodium or potassium salts, can be made available separately to be omitted or added in modified amounts in the final formulation given to the patient.

A number of reports have appeared in the literature and advertising concerning the usefulness of such commercial defined formula diets in a variety of clinical situations. While there are supporting data for the value of such formulations in certain situations with specific types of patients, the data are often not definitive. It is recommended that the physician and dietitian maintain an objective and questioning attitude in this area until they gain more experience with formulations in the treatment of specific diseases and more data are available. The patient who has no impaired digestion or absorption, but who for one reason or another has to be fed by tube, does not need special and expensive defined formulations, but rather food dispersed in water. The decision as to which nutritionally complete formula is most desirable for that patient should be based upon

1. total requirements for fluids, sodium, and other nutrients,
2. cost,
3. ease of preparation, and
4. the ability of the formula to flow through the feeding tube.

Decisions relating to frequency and rate of feeding will depend on the clinical situation. When there is known malabsorption, one should not accept *a priori* the concept that a formula with intact protein will be less well absorbed than one with hydrolysate or free amino acids or that a diet containing fat or polysaccharides is inferior to one without fat or with oligosaccharides.

Where there is significant malabsorption because of damaged or absent small intestine, the overall capacity of the remaining bowel to absorb will bear a relation not only to the composition of the formulation but also to the rate and the duration of time during which food is flowing past the available total absorbing surface area. If food is given rapidly in large volume, digestive enzymes will have a more limited opportunity to digest the large bulk of the formula before it has moved past the absorbing surface. The bolus feeding also greatly reduces the duration of exposure of the absorbing cells to the nutrients available for absorption. In such a situation slow infusion of formula by tube for prolonged periods (24 hours per day if necessary) will allow significantly more absorption than will bolus feeding. It also follows that a diet with constituents such as intact protein, fat, and polysaccharides, which might be inadequate for the patient when given in bolus fashion, could be quite adequate to maintain or improve nutrition if fed slowly.

When malabsorption is severe there is theoretical, and perhaps actual, advantage in initially infusing "predigested" formulations. These would contain hydrolyzed protein or free amino acids, oligosaccharides, and little or no fat to eliminate the need for the finite time of digestion of intact protein and polysaccharides by pancreatic enzymes and of long chain fats requiring lipase and conjugated bile salts. There is increasing experimental evidence for more rapid absorption of certain dipeptides and tripeptides than of free amino acids by normal intestinal epithelium (17) but the significance of these observations for optimum formula composition in treating serious malabsorption is still unknown. Oligosaccharides are hydrolyzed to glucose by the brush border enzyme, sucrase-α-dextrinase (18). Because of longer chain lengths, their use in formulas decreases osmolality significantly below that of equal amounts of monosaccharides or disaccharides. However, it is possible that mixtures of oligosaccharides, disaccharides, and monosaccharides may be more efficiently absorbed. There are very few data available on comparative absorption studies using different types of defined formula diets.

The need for maximizing nutrient and fluid absorption in patients with serious malabsorption is accentuated when portions of colon are also absent or damaged, since diarrhea will be intensified. Close attention to fluid and electrolyte requirements becomes even more essential. Magnesium depletion is particularly likely to develop in such individuals.

Of special interest in cancer patients is the actual or potential value of defined formula diets in the following areas:

1. in ameliorating intestinal epithelial damage induced by chemotherapeutic agents and radiation; this is a subject with contradictory evidence and requires further study,
2. in minimizing pancreatic secretion in pancreatitis and pancreatic fistula,
3. in the treatment of fistulas of the alimentary tract,
4. in maintaining or stimulating intestinal epithelial mass and function, and
5. in the treatment of organ failure.

These aspects have recently been reviewed (8).

Forced Feeding and Tumor Growth

Experience indicates that the great majority of patients with active malignancies can be rehabilitated nutritionally with tube feedings as well as with total parenteral nutrition. It is a rare patient who has obvious and rapid growth of tumor during repletion. However, this does not mean that residual tumor is not growing in conjunction with improved nutrition. For those patients undergoing prolonged nutritional therapy for various reasons who are known or suspected to have residual tumor, consideration should be given to concomitant adequate courses of antitumor therapy where there is no contraindication.

REFERENCES

1. E. M. MacCarthy-Leventhal, *Lancet* **2**, 1138 (1959).
2. M. E. Shils, *Surg. Gynecol. Obstet.* **132**, 709 (1971).
3. J. A. Williams, *Brit. Med. J.* **4**, 403; 467 (1967).
4. H. S. Hillman, *Gut* **9**, 576 (1968).
5. M. Miyata, T. Takao, T. Uozumi, E. Okamoto, and H. Manabe, *Ann. Surg.* **179**, 494 (1974).
6. R. Garrick, A. W. Ireland, and S. Posen, *Ann. Intern. Med.* **75**, 221, (1971); J. F. Adams, J. M. Johnstone, and R. D. Hunter, *Lancet* **1**, 415, (1960).
7. J. G. Fortner, *Surgery* **73**, 307 (1973).
8. M. E. Shils, *Cancer Res.,* in press.
9. N. F. La Russo, M. G. Korman, N .E. Hoffman, and A. F. Hofmann, *New Engl. J. Med.,* **291**, 690 (1974).
10. J. Q. Stauffer, M. H. Humphreys, and G. J. Weir, *Ann. Intern. Med.* **79**, 383 (1973); J. W. Dobbins and H. J. Binder, *Gastroenterology* **70**, 1096 (1976).
11. E. Weser, *Gastroenterology* **71**, 146 (1976).
12. M. E. Shils, *Am. J. Clin. Nutr.* **28**, 1429 (1975).

13. B. Langer, J. D. McHattie, W. J. Zohrab, and K. N. Jeejeebhoy, *J. Surg. Res.* **15**, 1973; J. W. Broviac and B. H. Scribner, *Surg. Gynecol. Obstet.* **139**, 24 (1974).

14. C. P. Page, J. A. Ryan, Jr., and R. C. Haff, *Surg. Gynecol. Obstet.* **142**, 184 (1976).

15. M. E. Shils, "Introduction to the Proc. Symp. Defined Formula Diets for Medical Use," Am. Med. Assoc., Chicago, in press.

16. M. E. Shils, A. S. Bloch, and R. Chernoff, *Clin. Bull. Memorial Hospital (NYC)* **6**, 151 (1976).

17. D. M. Matthews, and S. A. Abidi, *Gastroenterology* **71**, 151 (1976).

18. G. M. Gray, *New Engl. J. Med.* **292**, 1225 (1975).

Index